AF740075

Therapeutic Embolization

Kiron Varghese • Srilakshmi Adhyapak

Therapeutic Embolization

Springer

Kiron Varghese
Department of Cardiology
St. John's Medical College Hospital
Bangalore
India

Srilakshmi Adhyapak
St. John's Medical College Hospital
Bangalore
India

ISBN 978-3-319-42492-7 ISBN 978-3-319-42494-1 (eBook)
DOI 10.1007/978-3-319-42494-1

Library of Congress Control Number: 2016956094

© Springer International Publishing Switzerland 2017
This work is subject to copyright. All rights are reserved by the Publisher, whether the whole or part of the material is concerned, specifically the rights of translation, reprinting, reuse of illustrations, recitation, broadcasting, reproduction on microfilms or in any other physical way, and transmission or information storage and retrieval, electronic adaptation, computer software, or by similar or dissimilar methodology now known or hereafter developed.
The use of general descriptive names, registered names, trademarks, service marks, etc. in this publication does not imply, even in the absence of a specific statement, that such names are exempt from the relevant protective laws and regulations and therefore free for general use.
The publisher, the authors and the editors are safe to assume that the advice and information in this book are believed to be true and accurate at the date of publication. Neither the publisher nor the authors or the editors give a warranty, express or implied, with respect to the material contained herein or for any errors or omissions that may have been made.

Printed on acid-free paper

This Springer imprint is published by Springer Nature
The registered company is Springer International Publishing AG Switzerland

Foreword

It is indeed a great pleasure writing a foreword for a book written by my colleague Dr. Kiron Varghese and his co-author, Dr. Srilakshmi A.

I have known Dr. Kiron Varghese for 16 years, and while working with him at St. John's Medical College Hospital, I always admired his cardiovascular interventional skills and his kindness and concern for patients. Apart from excelling in coronary interventions, he evinced a keen interest in peripheral vascular interventions, rather an "orphaned field" those days. I watched him doing a bronchial artery embolization and salvaging a patient with massive hemoptysis getting almost drowned in his own secretions. Then onwards, he extended his field and expanded indications progressing forward, with gratifying results with therapeutic embolizations. Literally and metaphorically, he has covered from head to foot most of the organs in his interventional work and all aspects of the procedures in his book.

Probably, this book is the first of its kind, creating a new field "therapeutic embolization" in cardiovascular interventions, involving emergency life-saving procedures and elective procedures, avoiding surgery in some cases, assisting surgeons in providing bloodless fields, embolizing unwanted and harmful organs, and chemoembolization. Dr. Kiron, assisted ably by Dr. Srilakshmi, a competent clinical cardiologist and academician, has encapsulated all his rich experience and work in this book.

This would be an extremely useful book for all the students of cardiology and for cardiovascular interventionists as well. The authors deserve to be congratulated on bringing out this book, and this book should find its rightful place in all medical libraries.

I wish the authors good luck and success.

Dr. S.S. Iyengar, DM(Cardiology), FRCP(E)
Manipal Hospital, Bangalore, 560017, India

Preface

The aim of this book is to provide cardiologists and radiologists a concise guide to vascular embolization. This book covers embolizations in various vascular beds, although intracranial embolizations have been excluded as this topic is in itself very vast, constituting material for a whole book or monograph.

This book is designed to provide a perspective to the operator regarding embolizations in various clinical settings. The indications, materials used, techniques, complications, and outcomes of embolization have been discussed in detail. This book does not claim to be a compendium or handbook of embolization. It is largely the work of the Editors and associates in this field. We wish to express our thanks to all the authors and publishers whose work has been mentioned in this book. We wish to especially thank Dr. C. Thomas Peter, Retired Director of Electrophysiology at Cedars Sinai Medical Center, Los Angeles, USA, for his constant encouragement and guidance.

Finally, we wish to thank the editorial and production staff of Springer for their professional help and cooperation in producing this book.

Bangalore, India

Kiron Varghese, MD, DM, FACC
Srilakshmi Adhyapak, DNB, DNB

Contents

Chapter 1
Overview of Vascular Embolizations: Indications, Complications and Guidelines

Abstract Therapeutic vascular embolization is a minimally invasive transcatheter procedure by which abnormal vasculature which is either congenital or a result of an acquired pathological process is obliterated, thereby resulting in clinical improvement. It has also been used for occlusion of normal vasculature to palliate neoplasms and ablate tissue. These normal or abnormal vessels either cause excessive bleeding or produce hemodynamic disturbances. This procedure has gained acceptance in terms of safety and efficacy with the advent of more advanced hardware like microcatheters, embolization materials and high resolution digital imaging. The rate of procedural complications is low with expanding operator expertise, making it the first line of treatment in several clinical situations reviewed in the following chapters.

Keywords Embolization • Vasculature • Capillary beds • Lesion • Infection

Introduction

The Society of Cardio Vascular Interventional Radiologists' standards of practice committee has established certain quality improvement guidelines for percutaneous transcatheter embolization [1]. It is recommended that the operator is involved in the follow-up of the patient for the success of the procedure. Close follow-up, with monitoring and management of the patient after the embolization procedure is appropriate for the operator.

The most important processes of care are (1) patient selection, (2) performing the procedure, and (3) monitoring the patient. The outcome measures or indicators for these processes are indications, success rates, and complication rates. Outcome measures are assigned threshold levels.

Percutaneous transcatheter embolization is defined as the intravascular deposition of particulate, liquid, or mechanical agents, or autologous blood clot to produce intentional vessel occlusion.

Embolic vascular occlusion may be performed at any level from large arteries or veins to the capillary beds, and it may be temporary or permanent in nature. Percutaneous transcatheter embolization may be undertaken with curative or palliative intent [2].

© Springer International Publishing Switzerland 2017

K. Varghese, S. Adhyapak, *Therapeutic Embolization*,
DOI 10.1007/978-3-319-42494-1_1

Embolization may be performed as a staged procedure, particularly incases of complex or multiple lesions. Successful embolization results in devascularization of a focal lesion or intentional reduction or cessation of blood flow to a target vascular bed or an entire organ.

Technical success reflects immediate results and is typically evaluated with completion angiography. **Clinical success** is based on the clinical outcome and complications in the 30 days immediately following the embolization procedure and is typically assessed by close patient follow-up. **Complete clinical success** is defined as the resolution of signs or symptoms that prompted the embolization procedure. **Partial clinical success** is defined as significant improvement of signs or symptoms after the procedure, with a positive impact on the clinical course of the patient and/or the subsequent need for re-intervention

Palliative embolization is considered successful if there is diminished symptomatology after the procedure (eg, decreased transfusion requirements following embolization of a malignancy).

The **target area** is defined as the focal lesion, vessel, vascular territory, or organ to be devascularized.

Target ischemia is defined as symptoms resulting from devascularization within the immediate vascular distribution of the target area. For example, the development of duodenal fibrosis and stenosis following gastro duodenal artery embolization.

Non-target embolization is defined as unintentional deposition of embolic material distant from the target area. For example, spinal artery embolization leading to paraplegia during bronchial artery embolization [3].

Stringent quality control guidelines have been framed for embolization procedures. Thresholds have been defined to indicate success rates and complications. When indicators of success rates fall below a minimum threshold and when complication rates go above a maximum threshold, a review should be performed to determine the cause of this and changes have to be implemented. Patient referral patterns and selection factors may dictate different threshold levels in different Institutions Therefore, universal thresholds cannot be set and individual minimum and maximum thresholds will need to be set.

Major complications are defined as those which result in sequelae leading to hospital admissions. These can be due to non-target embolization like paraplegia. It can also be the result of excessive embolization leading to tissue necrosis and abscess formation.

Minor complications are those that do not result in sequelae. These can be the post-embolization syndrome of fever and leukocytosis.

Procedural Complications

Complication rates are heavily dependent on operator experience, vascular territory, the specific lesion addressed, and on the clinical condition of the patient. Patients with hemodynamic instability, multi-organ failure, malignancies, coagulopathy, renal failure, and infection tend to have higher complication rates.

Infectious complication scan be minimized by antibiotic prophylaxis and pneumoccal vaccination in patients undergoing splenic embolization and in cases in which bacterial contamination is likely (e.g., colon, open trauma, and some hepatic embolizations).

The embolization procedure should always be documented by completion angiography. Incomplete embolization may leave the patient exposed to the risks that the procedure was intended to alleviate [4]. In addition, in some preoperative cases incomplete embolization may increase the risk of operative hemorrhage [5]. Incomplete embolization also has been reported to cause hemolysis.

The indications for vascular embolization have been laid out as,

1. Occlusion of congenital or acquired vascular abnormalities, (e.g., aneurysm, pseudoaneurysm, arteriovenous fistula, arteriovenous formation and hemangioma) [4, 6–22].
2. Treatment of acute or recurrent hemorrhage (e.g., hemoptysis, gastrointestinal bleeding, posttraumatic and iatrogenic hemorrhage, and hemorrhagic neoplasms) [23].
3. Devascularization of neoplasms for palliation or to reduce operative blood loss [5, 24, 25].
4. Ablation of non-neoplastic tissue that produces adverse health effects to the patient (e.g., hypersplenism, refractory renovascular hypertension, proteinuria, urineleak, varicocele, pelvic congestion syndrome, priapism, and abdominal pregnancy) [26–37].
5. Flow redistribution to protect normal tissue (e.g., hepatic artery chemoembolization or proximal superior gluteal artery embolization in therapy for pelvic hemorrhage) [38, 39].

The decision to perform percutaneous transcatheter embolization should be made after considering the risks and benefits to each patient. Coagulopathy, sepsis, and renal failure are relative contraindications to percutaneous transcatheter embolization. Appropriate efforts should be made to correct or improve these conditions prior to the procedure. Lack of safe access to the target is another contraindication to treatment.

Stable catheter position may not be achieved in a minority of patients which could increase the risk of non target embolisation.

In other patients, a vascular communication may exist between the target and an adjacent vital structure (e.g., spinal arteries arising from bronchial, intercostal, or lumbar vessels). This has been viewed as an absolute contraindication by some authors and as a relative contraindication by others [40–42].

Published rates for individual types of complications are highly dependent on patient selection and are based on series comprising several 100 patients, which is a number larger than most individual practitioners are likely to treat. It is also recognized that a single complication can cause a rate to cross above a complication-specific threshold when the complication occurs in a small volume of patients. In this situation, the overall procedure threshold is more appropriate for use.

References

1. Drooz AT, Lewis CA, Allen TE, Citron SJ, Cole PE, Freeman NJ, Husted JW, Malloy PC, Martin LG, Van Moore A, Neithamer CD, Roberts AC, Sacks D, Sanchez O, Venbrux AC, Sakal CW, SCVIR Standards of Practice Committee. Quality improvement guidelines for percutaneous transcatheter embolization. J Vasc Interv Radiol. 1997;8:889–95.
2. Cox GG, Lee KR, Price HI, Gunter K, Noble J, Mebust WK. Colonic infarction following ethanol embolization of renal-cell carcinoma. Radiology. 1982;145:343–5.
3. Gang DL, Dole KB, Adelman LS. Spinal cord infarction following therapeutic renal artery embolization. JAMA. 1977;237:2841–2.
4. Onohara T, Okadome K, Mii S, Yasumori K, Muto Y, Sugimachi K. Rupture of embolised coeliac artery pseudoaneurysm into the stomach: is coil embolisation an effective treatment for coeliac anastomotic pseudoaneurysm? Eur J Vasc Surg. 1992;6:330–2.
5. Bakal CW, Cynamon J, Lakritz PS, Sprayregen S. Value of preoperative renal artery embolization in reducing blood transfusion requirements during nephrectomy for renal cell carcinoma. J Vasc Interv Radiol. 1993;4:727–31.
6. Gabata T, Matsui O, Nakamura Y, Kimura M, Tsuchiyama T, Takashima T. Transcatheter embolization of traumatic mesenteric hemorrhage. J Vasc Interv Radiol. 1994;5:891–4.
7. Mauro MA, Jaques P. Transcatheter management of pseudoaneurysms complicating pancreatitis. J Vasc Interv Radiol. 1991;2:527–32.
8. Baker KS, Tisnado J, Cho SR, Beachley MC. Splanchnic artery aneurysms and pseudoaneurysms: transcatheter embolization. Radiology. 1987;163:135–9.
9. Keller FS, Rosch J, Baur GM, Taylor LM, Dotter CT, Porter JM. Percutaneous angiographic embolization: a procedure of increasing usefulness. Am J Surg 1981;142:5–11.
10. Stanley P, Grinnell V, Stanton RE, Williams KO, Shore NA. Therapeutic embolization of infantile hepatic hemangioma with polyvinyl alcohol. AJR Am J Roentgenol. 1983;141:1047–51.
11. Goldblatt M, Goldin AR. Percutaneous embolization for the management of hepatic artery aneurysms. Gastroenterology. 1977;73:1142–6.
12. Hollis Jr HW, Luethke JM, Yakes WF, Beitler AL. Percutaneous embolization of an internal ilia cartery aneurysm: technical considerations and literature review. J Vasc Interv Radiol. 1994;5:449–51.
13. Beller U, Rosen RJ, Beckman EM, Markoff G, Berenstein A. Congenital arteriovenous malformation of the female pelvis: a gynecologic perspective. Am J Obstet Gynecol. 1988;159:1153–60.
14. Abbas FM, Currie JL, Mitchell S, Osterman F, Rosenshein NB, Horowitz IR. Selective vascular embolization in benign gynecologic conditions. J Reprod Med. 1994;39:492–6.
15. Komoda K, Hujii Y, Nakajima T, et al. A ruptured thymic branch aneurysm mimicking a ruptured aortic aneurysm, with associated bronchial artery aneurysms: report of a case. Jpn J Surg. 1994;24:258262.
16. Remy-Jardin M, Wattinne L, Remy J. Transcatheter occlusion of pulmonary arterial circulation and collateral supply: failures, incidents and complications. Radiology. 1991;180:699–705.
17. Boudghene F, L'Hermine C, Bigot JM. Arterial complications of pancreatitis: diagnostic and therapeutic aspects in 104 cases. J Vasc Interv Radiol. 1993;4:551–8.
18. Kadir S, Marshall FF, White Jr RI, Kaufman SL, Barth KH. Therapeutic embolization of the kidney with detachable silicone balloons. J Urol. 1983;129:11–3.
19. Eckstein MR, Waltman AC, Athanasoulis CA. Interventional angiography of the renal fossa. Radiol Clin North Am. 1984;22:381–92.
20. Mazer MJ, Baltaxe HA, Wolf GL. Therapeutic embolization of the renal artery with Gianturco coils: limitations and technical pitfalls. Radiology. 1981;138:37–46.
21. White Jr RI, Lynch-Nyhan A, Terry P, et al. Pulmonary arteriovenous malformations: techniques and long-term outcome of embolo therapy. Radiology. 1988;169:663–9.

22. Hemingway AP, Allison DJ. Complications of embolization: analysis of 410 procedures. Radiology. 1988;166:669–72.
23. Cohen AM, Antoun BW, Stern RC. Left thyrocervical trunk bronchial artery supplying right lung: source of recurrent hemoptysis in cysticfibrosis. AJR Am J Roentgenol. 1992;158:1131–3.
24. O'Keeffe FN, Carrasco CH, Charnsangavej C, Richli WR, Wallace S. Arterial embolization of adrenal tumors: results in nine cases. AJR Am J Roentgenol. 1988;151:819–922.
25. Kennelly MJ, Grossman HB, Cho KJ. Outcome analysis of 42 cases of renal angiomyolipoma. J Urol. 1994;152:1988–91.
26. McLean GK, Meranze SG. Embolization techniques in the urinary tract. Radiol Clin North Am. 1986;24:671–82.
27. Spigos DG, Jonasson O, Mozes M, Capek V. Partial splenic embolization in the treatment of hypersplenism. AJR Am J Roentgenol. 1979;132:777–82.
28. Kerr A, Trambert J, Mikhail M, Hodges L, Runowicz C. Preoperative transcatheter embolization of abdominal pregnancy: report of three cases. J Vasc Interv Radiol. 1993;4:733–5.
29. Reyes BL, Trerotola SO, Venbrux AC, et al. Percutaneous embolo therapy of adolescent varicocele: results and long-term follow-up. J Vasc Interv Radiol. 1994;5:131–4.
30. Porst H, Bahren W, Lenz M, Altwein JE. Percutaneous sclerotherapy of varicoceles: an alternative to conventional surgical methods. Br J Urol. 1984;56:73–8.
31. Zuckerman AM, Mitchell SE, Venbrux AC, et al. Percutaneous varicocele occlusion: long-term follow-up. J Vasc Interv Radiol. 1994;5:315–9.
32. Morag B, Rubinstein ZJ, Goldwasser B, Yerushalmi A, Lunnenfeld B. Percutaneous venography and occlusion in the management of spermatic varicoceles. AJR Am J Roentgenol. 1984;143:635–40.
33. Hunter DW, King III NJ, Aeppli DM, et al. Spermatic vein occlusion with hot contrast material: angiographic results. J Vasc Interv Radiol. 1991;2:507–15.
34. Wernovsky G, Bridges ND, Mandell VS, Castaneda AR, Perry SB. Enlarged bronchial arteries after early repair of transposition of the great arteries. J Am Coll Cardiol. 1993;21:465–70.
35. Spigos DG, Tan WS, Mozes MF, Pringle K, Iossifides I. Splenic embolization. Cardiovasc Intervent Radiol. 1980;3:282–8.
36. Keller FS, Coyle M, Rosch J, Dotter CT. Percutaneous renal ablation in patients with end-stage renal disease: alternative to surgical nephrectomy. Radiology. 1986;159:447–51.
37. Machan LS. Gynecologic interventional radiology. Presented at the 21st annual scientific meeting of the Society of Cardiovascular and Interventional Radiology, March 27, 1996, Seattle.
38. Feldman L, Greenfield AJ, Waltman AC. Transcatheter vessel occlusion: angiographic results versus clinical success. Radiology. 1983;147:1–5.
39. Chuang VP, Wallace S, Gianturco C, Soo CS. Complications of coil embolization: prevention and management. AJR Am J Roentgenol. 1981;137:809–13.
40. Uflacker R, Kaemmerer A, Neves C, Picon PD. Management of massive hemoptysis by bronchial artery embolization. Radiology. 1983;146:627–34.
41. Uflacker R, Kaemmerer A, Picon PD, et al. Bronchial artery embolization in the management of hemoptysis: technical aspects and long-term results. Radiology. 1985;157:637–44.
42. Miller FJ, Mineau DE. Transcatheter arterial embolization: major complications and their prevention. Cardiovasc Intervent Radiol. 1983;6:141–9.

Chapter 2
Materials Used for Vascular Embolization

Abstract Therapeutic embolization requires the use of materials which are stable and of sufficient caliber to embolize the specific vascular structure. Hence, in smaller vessels which need embolization, smaller particles or liquid materials may be required. PolyVinyl Alcohol particles and Gel Foam have been used with success. Coils of varying diameters have been used for embolization of large caliber vasculature. Successful embolization has been defined as sluggish flow to total absence of flow distal to the site of embolization. Here, the properties and indications of various embolization materials have been discussed.

Keywords Embolization • Poly Vinyl Alcohol • Coils

Introduction

Gel foam and Poly Vinyl Alcohol (PVA) particles have been used for therapeutic embolization in the bronchial arterial bed and in certain arterio-venous malformations. These are more suited for embolization of small caliber vessels. Large caliber vessels for embolization require coils and vascular devices.

Properties of Gel Foam and PVA Particles

Gel Foam is easy to use since it slides smoothly through most catheters when the particles are suspended in contrast material or non-contrast aqueous fluids (Fig. 2.1). However, it is not an ideal agent as it gets fairly quickly degraded by the body's proteolytic enzymes permitting rapid recanalization of embolized vessels.

PVA particles take months to years to get absorbed by the body [1], and are considered effectively permanent. They have a high coefficient of friction which cause the individual particles to roll within the embolization catheter resulting in " log-jams. " Although this can be overcome by simply increasing the force of injection,

© Springer International Publishing Switzerland 2017
K. Varghese, S. Adhyapak, *Therapeutic Embolization*,
DOI 10.1007/978-3-319-42494-1_2

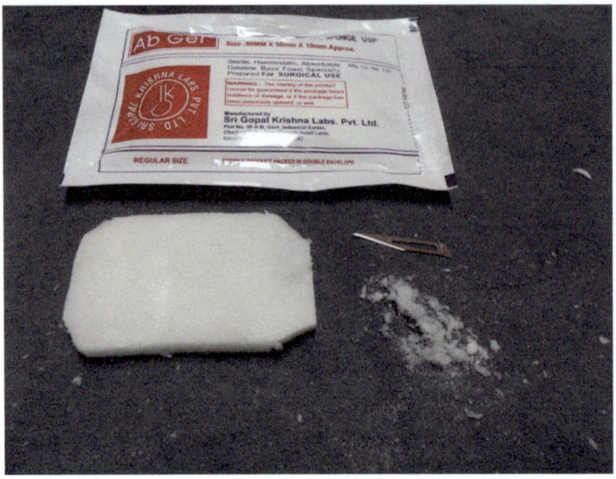

Fig. 2.1 Gelfoam material which is used for embolization after shaving off fine particles from it with a scalpel blade. These particles are mixed with contrast and saline mixture

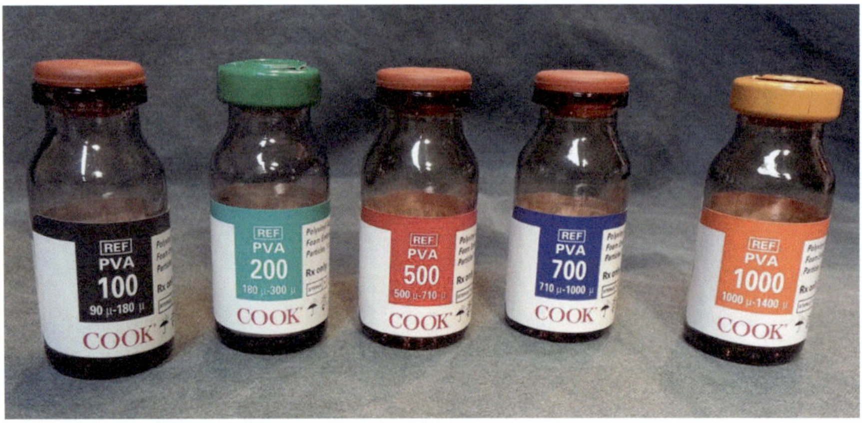

Fig. 2.2 PVA particles in sizes of 100 µ, 200 µ, 500 µ and 700 µ. These are mixed with contrast and saline mixture before injecting into the target vessel to be embolized

it cannot usually be done with maintenance of the physiologic " slowflow" technique [2].

Gelfoam has little frictional drag, the particles flow smoothly within the catheter with little rotation.

PVA particle passage is more complex (Fig. 2.2). Having a much higher coefficient of friction, PVA particles tend to tumble. So long as all PVA particles are the same size and shape and, most importantly, are very widely spaced, they move almost as easily as Gelfoam. But they suspend much less well than do Gelfoam particles as their shape is irregular, and the particles tend to jam with greater frequency when used in usual concentrations (Fig. 2.3).

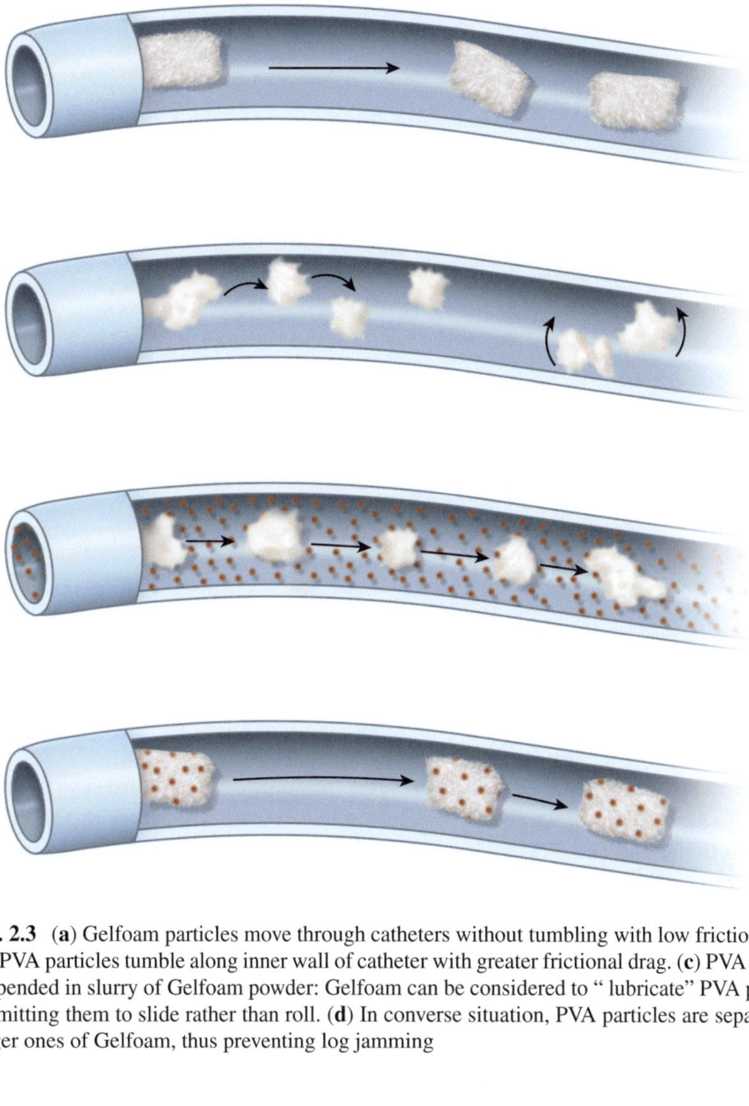

Fig. 2.3 (**a**) Gelfoam particles move through catheters without tumbling with low frictional drag. (**b**) PVA particles tumble along inner wall of catheter with greater frictional drag. (**c**) PVA particles suspended in slurry of Gelfoam powder: Gelfoam can be considered to " lubricate" PVA particles, permitting them to slide rather than roll. (**d**) In converse situation, PVA particles are separated by larger ones of Gelfoam, thus preventing log jamming

PVA Particles

These particles are generally elliptical and are assumed to be lying flat on a surface when they are measured. The actual minor axis will usually be the unmeasured vertical height of the particle, whereas the actual intermediate axis will be approximated by the measured minor axis [6, 15]. The minimum measured axis will therefore be a conservative estimation of the intermediate axis; it will range in value between the actual minor and intermediate axes. The ability of a particle to pass through a given sieve dimension primarily depends on its intermediate axis, so the mean minimum axis is the determined size (Fig. 2.4). Knowledge of particle

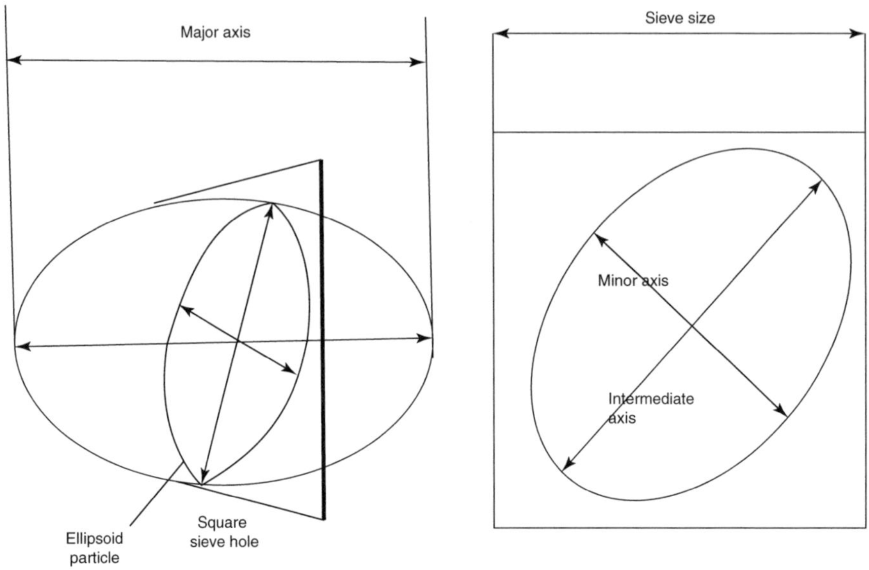

Fig. 2.4 Diagram of a hypothetical particle passing through a square sieve hole. The major axis lines up perpendicular to the plane of the sieve in the lateral view (**a**). The minor and intermediate axis are shown from above in (**b**). The major and minor axes do not determine the particle's ability to pass through the sieve as much as the intermediate axis

uniformity and size is vital for several reasons. A specific combination of catheter diameter and particle size is selected for each embolization procedure. The catheter must be flexible and small enough to allow selective catheterization of the vessel supplying the lesion and yet be large enough to deliver embolic agents. The particles must fit through the catheter without causing catheter occlusion yet not be so small that they pass through the circulation of the lesion. The selection of the optimal combination of catheter diameter and particle size therefore requires an accurate knowledge of particle dimensions and uniformity. Larger particles are more likely to occlude the catheter and smaller particles are less likely to cause successful embolization.

Combinations of Gel Foam and PVA particles have been used in certain situations where ease of use combined with longer permanence is required. Embolization of abnormalities proximal to capillary beds (e.g., vascular tumors) can be accomplished with a mixture of PVA particles and Gelfoam suspended in contrast material. High-flow lesions (e.g., arteriovenous malformations), which do not provide the protective filtering action of capillary beds, may require larger Gelfoam particles mixed with smaller sizes of PVA. Each of these combinations should have the advantages of both ease of use and relative permanence.

The combination of Gel Foam and PVA particles has been used to embolize Intra-cranial arterio-venous malformations (AVM). Dural and pial AVM s have been embolized with no recurrence due to re canalization [AJNR]. The feeders to the AVM from the external carotid artery were embolized. A facial hemangioma involving the maxilla and mandible was embolized with clinical resolution. After embolization of a pheochromocytoma, catecholamines were found to be decreased to 8 % of pre-embolization values. Renal artery embolization was done with this mixture for a renal tumor making transection of the renal artery and vein during nephrectomy, almost bloodless. Embolization of an extremity tumor rendered about 100 ml of blood loss during resection. This was despite the fact that surgery was necessarily performed too proximally to permit use of a tourniquet. Dissection of the mass from surrounding tissue was reported by the orthopedic surgeons to have been facilitated by devascularization of the tumor.

PVA-Gelfoam mixture permits the luxury of a planned stabilization interval between embolization and surgery without concern that the occlusion and additional thrombosis will be resorbed. Although permanent endovascular occlusion with PVA is unreliable, solid occlusion has been found to persist long enough to kill tissue. Histology of the biopsy specimens show a constant occurrence of disruption of the internal elastic lamina. Only occasional giant cells are seen. A combination of both Gel Foam and PVA particles helps overcome the disadvantages of the individual agents and may be more efficacious [5, 14].

Detachable Balloons

Detachable balloons used to be used for embolization which has declined in the past few years. There are several reasons for the same, mainly advances in other permanent embolization materials and lack of developmental attention to them by the medical device industry. The delivery systems of large guiding catheters was also less desirable. Placement was flow directed with very little steerability [16–18].

They consist of a balloon inflation delivery catheter and an introducer catheter. The balloons are made of either latex or silicone. The silicone balloons are more stable and not as degradable as latex. Filling the silicone balloon with iso-osmolar contrast is important for long lasting inflation. Hypo-osmolar contrast may cause balloon deflation and recanalization of the blood vessel. The latex balloons are not dependent on osmolarity, however they may cause vascular recanalization which is related to latex degradation or leaking of the valve mechanism. Vascular embolization occurs successfully if the balloon remains inflated for atleast 3 weeks.

The disadvantages and pitfalls are plenty. Early detachment is a concern, especially when deploying through a co-axial catheter. Post-deployment migration is another concern, especially when it is not sized appropriately to the target vessel. Certain anatomic and physiologic characteristics may also predispose to balloon migration. A sharply tapered vessel will have a tendency to expel the balloon. Compliant vessels may enlarge in diameter in response to respiratory excursions or in response to the occlusion, as greater hemodynamic forces are transmitted to the wall. Further drag forces in high flow vessels and arterio-venous fistulae can cause balloon elongation. With poor traction against the wall, the balloon may embolize distally or may reflux into the parent vessel and embolize elsewhere.

Difficulty in detaching a balloon may also occur due to geometric, anatomic or physiologic factors. If this occurs, controlled deflation and removal may be necessary.

These have been removed from the US market due to its potential migration issues.

Coil Emboli

These are the most widely used mechanical emboli. First described by Gianturco, the coil was 3 mm long 19 gauge piece of steel tubing with cotton threads attached to it. The second device was a 5 cms long coiled piece of 0.038 in. steel guide wire with its central mandril core removed and four 3 cms long woolen strands attached to its tip. This was introduced into a non tapered 7 F Teflon catheter using a thin mandril extending from the 19 gauge steel tubing. It is then advanced through the catheter using a 0.045 or 0.052 in. guidewire. Early experience demonstrated complete vascular occlusion of the target vasculature, although multiple coils were required for larger vessel embolization. While metal and fabric created physical occlusion of the vessel, complete occlusion was due to thrombus formation. Late recanalization was rare [7, 9].

Over the years, several refinements have led to the development of thinner coils permitting their delivery through 3 F catheters or smaller catheters. Wool has been replaced by Dacron which causes a less severe inflammatory reaction in the vessel wall.

The size of the coils can be 0.034–0.038 in. for delivery through a 5 F catheter and 0.018 in. through a 3 F microcatheter. Small vessels can be approached by co-axial microcatheters. In addition to allowing super-selective distal catheterization, when used with soft, steerable wires cause less spasm. The smaller coils can be delivered through them using 0.018 in. soft glidewires, which are special coil pushers or by forceful saline flushes. The larger coils can be delivered through larger catheters which are co-axial to the target vessel using steerable guidewires to push them into place. Occasionally, the first portion of the first coil can be anchored in a side branch to prevent coil migration [7].

Coils are made of stainless steel, platinum and nitinol with Dacron strands attached to them. Helical diameters of 3–15 mm and lengths of 2–15 cms are available. Platinum coils have technical advantages over stainless steel in that they are softer and can be compressed into tighter coils and cause lesser vessel injury. They have Dacron fibers aiding in thrombogenicity. Macrocoils and microcoils are available. Nester coils are 0.035–0.038 in. and are helically shaped. Tornado coils are 0.035 in. and are conical in shape. Hilal coils are 0.018 in. and are intended for super-selective embolization. Nitinol in addition has certain properties of 'thermal shape memory' and prevents herniation of additional coils deployed into the parent artery.

Coil Deployment

Deployment falls into two categories, pushable and detachable. Pushable coils are most frequently used in peripheral interventions. They consist of a pre-loaded, elongated coil inserted into a catheter. Once inserted, the coil can be advanced into position by a coil pusher or a guidewire. Alternately, a forcible saline injection can be used to deliver the coil into position.

Detachable coils employ the twist mechanism. The coil is attached to a twistable delivery wire which is twisted when the coil is in the right position for embolization. This is used for neurovascular embolizations, congenital heart diseases, especially in the setting of aorto-pulmonary fistulae.

Technicalities of Coil Embolization

Adequate scaffolding should be obtained by initially deploying a larger coil, followed by smaller ones.

An Amplatzer Vascular Obstruction Device can be used for vessels that do not taper as it has legs that can penetrate the walls of the vessel, acting as a cone into which coils may be placed.

In patients with coagulopathies as in situations of trauma/shock, coils can be used as a scaffold in combination with Gelfoam such a "coil-Gelfoam sandwich" causes a complete, permanent mechanical occlusion. Stiffer coils are generally deployed first and are used as a "backstop." Softer and pliable coils with unpredictable coil shapes that tend to conform to vessel anatomy, such as the Nestor coil (Cook, Inc.,Bloomington, IN), may be deployed following a stiffer "backstop" coil deployment. Microcatheters should be used when the coil is <0.018 in. (microcoil) to prevent catheter occlusion. Care should be taken to be certain that "high-flow" catheters are used with caution when deploying coils, as the larger inner lumen may allow the coils to partially form in the catheter, leading to catheter blockage. Undersizing of the coil may lead to distal embolization and must be avoided especially in cases of pulmonary artery AVM. As a rule of thumb, the coil should be 20 % larger than the vessel diameter.

Too much oversizing of the coil will prevent the coil from achieving its shape, leading to inadequate occlusions, as well as a markedly longer coil (which may in turn lead to proximal coil malposition).

When deployment precision is required (i.e., intracranial procedures, PAVM), coils may be deployed using the floppy end of a "pusher wire"; when precision of deployment is not a concern (i.e., filling a pseudoaneurysm), the coil may be deployed using a saline bolus.

Retrievable coils allow the coil to be pulled back in the delivery catheter just before deployment. This technique is also helpful when precise placement is essential [8].

As a rule of thumb, steel coils tend to be stiffer while platinum coils tend to be softer.

Amplatzer Vascular Plug

A self-expandable device made of nitinol mesh, Amplatzer Vascular Plugs are used when a permanent large vessel occlusion is required. Initially composed of a single biconcave disc, the current device is composed of three adjacent discs connected to one another. This stacked configuration leads to a more rapid and complete vessel occlusion. Devices are available ranging from 4 to 16 mm in diameter.

The device should be oversized by 15–30 % (30–50 % for the single disc device) relative to the vessel to prevent distal migration. It has two platinum bands which serve as radiopaque markers for optimal positioning. A simple unscrewing mechanism allows for precise deployment of the device.

Guide Wires

Movable core guide wires are used freserved for very large aneurysms and pseudoaneurysms. The outer coiled spring with Teflon wrapping is the part of the guide wire used for embolization. The inner mandril and safety wire are discarded. Guide wires offer little to no thrombogenic potential, but rather are used as a cheap and easy method to "take up space" in a very large vascular space.

Repositioning the wires is extremely difficult. Once deployed, the wires tend to conform to the outer contour of the aneurysm while the inner portion of the sac remains patent. Guide wires by themselves are generally insufficient for complete thrombosis, and combination with other devices is generally necessary.

Suture Material

Sutures may be used in conjunction with other agents. 2–0 or 3–0 silk suture is cut into 5- to 10-mm pieces prior to embolization. The suture fragments are delivered hydrostatically by injecting with a 1- to 3-mL syringe. Sutures are radiolucent, and therefore the use of a syringe filled with contrast for injection followed by a saline flush is necessary. Hydrostatic deployment confers little to no control, making non-target embolization a distinct possibility. Hence, this embolization material is no longer in use.

Before choosing an embolic agent, it is necessary for the operator to address the following questions,

1. How large is the vessel to be embolized? Any vessel that can be seen angiographically is considered large. Vessels smaller than the resolution of digital subtraction angiography are considered small.
2. How long should the vessel remain occluded following embolization? Temporary occlusion implies occlusion of the vessel for hours to weeks; permanent occlusion is self-explanatory.
3. Should the embolized tissue remain viable after embolization? Ischemia is often a result (intended or unintended) of embolization. Intentional organ or cellular death implies using specific embolic agents.

Large-Vessel Permanent Occlusion

Clinical scenarios in which large-vessel permanent occlusion is required are situations in which angiographically visualized vascular abnormalities are present and a therapeutic permanent occlusion of these abnormalities is required. In these situations, the end organ supplied by the embolized vessel has a good collateral blood supply, preventing organ death following successful embolization. For this purpose, coils and Amplatzer plugs are the usual embolic agents used. Such a proximal large-vessel occlusion is the equivalent of surgical ligation of the vessel.

Large-Vessel Temporary Occlusion

Clinical scenarios in which a large-vessel temporary occlusion is desired are situations where temporary arrest of hemorrhage is necessary with subsequent recanalization and vessel healing. In these situations, Gelfoam sponge is used, either as a slurry or torpedoes [3, 4].

Small Vessel Embolization

The smaller the agent, the greater is the likelihood of organ ischemia. Most organs have some duplication of vascular supply; this collateralization is vital to organ survival following a proximal vascular event. If very small embolic agents are used, the effective level of the embolization is distal to where the collateral vessels join the main feeding artery, thereby effectively occluding inflow from both the primary and collateral circulations. Therefore, for most organ systems, small agents cause much greater ischemia than larger agents [13].

Particles

PolyVinyl Alcohol particles are generally used and range from 45 to 1180 mm in diameter.

Frequent agitation or addition of albumin (rarely used today) may prevent clumping, which is a common problem due to PVA's natural buoyancy. Particle size should be matched to the delivery catheter used to prevent catheter occlusion (generally microcatheters are used for particles <700 mm). Forceful injection during the procedure may result in reflux of particles into a nontarget vessel due to "explosive" delivery.

Trisacryl Microspheres

Trisacryl microspheres or embospheres are also used for vascular embolization. They are non resorbable and hydrophilic particles made from an acrylic polymer matrix combined with porcine gelatin. They are available in 20 ml prefilled syringes containing embospheres of various sizes : 40 to 120 mm, 100 to 300 mm, 300 to 500 mm, 500 to 700 mm, 700 to 900 mm, and 900 to 1200 mm.

In contrast to PVA particles which are irregular in shape and tend to aggregate within the hub or shaft of the delivery catheter, embospheres are spherical, smooth, precisely calibrated and non-resorbable hydrophilic particles and less likely to cause occlusion of the catheter.

As with PVA particles, the syringes containing the embospheres need to be agitated intermittently in order to maintain them in suspension and prevent aggregation or sedimentation. In addition, embospheres have allergic potential due to the inclusion of porcine gelatin. While embospheres may penetrate more deeply into the vascular beds and have superior clinical outcomes compared with PVA they may also cause unintended ischemia is some vascular beds.

Liquid Embolic Agents

Cyanoacrylates (glue) are tissue adhesive materials that polymerize rapidly once exposed to an ionic environment such as saline or blood, forming a cast of the vessel in which polymerization occurs. Ethiodol (Savage Laboratories, Melville, NY) is mixed with the glue to render cyanoacrylate radiopaque.

Ethylene Vinyl Alcohol Copolymer (Onyx) Liquid Embolic System (Micro Therapeutics, Plymouth, MN) is a foam like adhesive substance that solidifies upon contact with ionic materials. Onyx solidifies from the periphery toward the center, resulting in a spongy substance that forms a cast of the vessel (e.g., the "skin" forms first, and the cast fills from the inside, analogous to filling a water balloon).

Cyanoacrylate Nonionic solutions must be used during preparation to prevent polymerization during delivery [11, 12].

To prevent catheter blockage, delivery catheter must be flushed with a nonionic solution, such as 5 % dextrose, before and after every use; separate "nonionic table" is usually set up; glove changes required before use; and immediate pre-use mixing are all helpful techniques to prevent catheter blockage.

For agents such as Ethylene-Vinyl Alcohol Copolymer (Onyx) Liquid Embolic System (Micro Therapeutics, Plymouth, MN), vials must be placed in a shaker for at least 20 min prior to the procedure, with continued agitation just prior to the delivery.

Sclerosants

Sclerosants are liquid embolization agents that produce nearly immediate and complete thrombosis and inflammation at the very small-vessel and tissue level. Knowledge of vascular anatomy and prevention of embolization to nontarget locations is of utmost importance. Absolute alcohol is extremely toxic to living tissues, leading to complete vessel thrombosis/occlusion as well as direct tissue ablation and cell death. Essentially, whatever alcohol touches, it kills. Sodium tetradecyl sulfate (1–3 %) is a mild sclerosant most often used for varicose vein, spermatic vein and renal ablations, pelvic congestion syndrome, and preoperative arteriovenous malformations. Boiling contrast has fallen out favor due to side effects (severe pain) [12].

Balloon inflation Balloon inflation proximal to the injection site and aggressive aspiration with a large syringe will prevent retrograde embolization. Contrast injection with an occlusion balloon inflated will help to estimate the volume of sclerosant needed. Patients usually sense an intense pain immediately after alcohol injection, and deep sedation or general anesthesia is usually recommended.

When using alcohol, a 4:1 mixture with lipiodol will render alcohol radiopaque.

Ethiodol is an inert oil-based contrast agent. Once injected, oil droplets break into smaller globules to 50 μm in diameter, leading to a distal functional-level embolization. Lipiodol has an affinity to hepatocellular carcinoma, increasing the selectivity of the embolization. Ethiodol (Savage Laboratories, Melville, NY) mixture ratio is used to modulate the polymerization time per operator's preference (1:1–1:6), with higher concentrations of lipiodol conferring prolonged polymerization times.

Powder Substances

There are numerous powder embolics. Gelfoam (Ethicon, Somerville, NJ) powder is supplied in 1-g aliquots of sterile powder with each particle measuring 50 mm. Like Gelfoam sponge, Gelfoam powder embolization results in temporary occlusion lasting from days to several weeks. Microfibrillated collagen (Avitene, Davol Inc.; Cranson, RI; Angiostat) is a temporary agent very similar to Gelfoam in its properties. It is available in both "sheet" (analogous to sponge) and "flour" (analogous to powder) forms, representing proximal and distal agents, respectively. Thrombin is a natural enzyme that converts fibrinogen to fibrin as one of the end steps in clot formation for both the intrinsic and extrinsic coagulation cascades. Thrombin is most often used for direct-puncture injection of postcatheterization pseudoaneurysms to facilitate thrombosis. It can also be used mixed with Gelfoam, for embolization of endoleaks following endovascular aneurysm repair. Starch microspheres are 50-mm porous spheres made of biodegradable starch that dissolve within minutes and are mainly utilized for distal small-artery temporary occlusion situations such as intra-arterial chemotherapy delivery [10].

Small Vessel Permanent Occlusion

In situations in which end-organ or tissue death is not acceptable or desired, such as some selective tumor embolizations, uterine fibroid embolization, bronchial artery embolization, or small vessel gastrointestinal bleeding, particles are typically used. As a rule of thumb, the larger the particle size, the less likely the risk of ischemia. Larger particles (>300 mm) are typically used in these patient populations [13].

In situations in which end-organ or tissue death is a desired end point, such as arteriovenous malformations, superselective tumor embolizations, and transcatheter renal ablation procedures, sclerosant liquid agents (absolute alcohol, sodium tetradecyl sulfate) and glues (cyanoacrylates, Onyx) are used. Ethiodol and thrombin may also be used as they cause occlusion at the very small-vessel level.

Small-Vessel Temporary Occlusion

This clinical situation is the least commonly encountered. Rarely used, small-vessel temporary occlusions may cause tissue ischemia but are designed to allow vessel recanalization. Such clinical settings typically involve tumor embolizations, where the operator knows that they are going to return for another round of treatment. Such agents include Gelfoam powder, starch microspheres, and Avitene.

Conclusions

By taking a standardized, structured approach to each clinical situation, the operator can usually choose an appropriate embolizing agent.

Asking the three simple questions outlined in this chapter as to the size of the vessel to be embolized, whether permanent or temporary occlusion is required, and whether organ death is desirable, will help the operator decide on the appropriate embolizing agent.

References

1. Porstman W, Wierny L, Wornke H, Gertberger G, Romonick PA. Catheter closure of patent ductus arteriosis. Radiol Clin North Am. 1971;9:203–18.
2. Kerber CW. Flow-controlled therapeutic embolization. A physiologic and safe technique. AJR Am J Roentgenol. 1980;134:557–61.
3. Bank WO, Kerber CW. Gelfoam embolization: a simplified technique. AJR Am J Roentgenol. 1979;132:299–301.
4. White Jr RI, Strandberg JV, Gross GS, Barth KH. Therapeutic embolization with long-term occluding agents and their effects on embolized tissues. Radiology. 1977;125:677–87.
5. Horton JA, Marano GD, Kerber CW, Jenkins JJ, Davis S. Polyvinyl alcohol foam-gel foam for therapeutic embolization: a synergistic mixture. AJNR Am J Neuroradiol. 1983;4:143–7.
6. Jack CR, Forbes G, Dewanjee MK, Brown ML, Earnest F. Polyvinyl alcohol sponge for embolotherapy: particle size and morphology. AJNR Am J Neuroradiol. 1985;6:595–7.
7. Bauer JR, Ray Jr CE. Embolization agents. In: Mauro M, Murphy K, Thomson K, Venbrux A, Zollikofer C, editors. Image- guided interventions. Philadelphia: Saunders Elsevier; 2008. p. 131–9.
8. Lubarsky M, Ray Jr CE, Funaki B. Embolization agents—which one should be used when? Part 1: large-vessel. Semin Interv Radiol. 2009;26:352–7.
9. Loffroy R, Guiu B, Cercueil JP, Krause' D. Endovascular therapeutic embolisation: an overview of occluding agents and their effects on embolised tissues. Curr Vasc Pharmacol. 2009;7:250–63.
10. Abada HT, Golzarian J. Gelatine sponge particles: handling characteristics for endovascular use. Tech Vasc Interv Radiol. 2007;10:257–60.
11. Laurent A. Microspheres and nonspherical particles for embolization. Tech Vasc Interv Radiol. 2007;10:248–56.
12. Howington JU, Kerber CW, Hopkins LN. Liquid embolic agents in the treatment of intracranial arteriovenous malformations. Neurosurg Clin N Am. 2005;16:355–63, ix–x.
13. Lubarsky M, Ray C, Funaki B. Embolization agents—which one should be used when? Part 2: small-vessel embolization. Semin Interv Radiol. 2010;27:99–104.
14. Horton JA, Marano GO, Kerber CW, Jenkins JJ, Oavis S. Polyvinyl alcohol foam-gelfoam for therapeutic embolization: a synergistic mixture. Am J Neuroradiol. 1983;4:143–7.
15. Derdeyn CP, Moran CJ, Cross DWT, Dietrich HH, Dacey Jr RG. Polyvinyl alcohol particle size and suspension characteristics. Am J Neuroradiol. 1995;16:1335–43.
16. White Jr RI, Barth KH, Kaufman SL, DeCaprio V, Strandberg JD. Therapeutic embolization with detachable balloons. Cardiovasc Intervent Radiol. 1980;3(4):229–41.
17. DeSouza NM, Reidy JF. Embolization with detachable balloons--applications outside the head. Clin Radiol. 1992;46(3):170–5.
18. Morris P. Detachable balloon embolization: safety balloon technique. Am J Neuroradiol. 2000;21:984.

Chapter 3
Bronchial Artery Embolization for Massive Hemoptysis

Abstract The most common devastating presenting symptom of patients with post-tubercular bronchiectasis of the lung is severe hemoptysis amounting to >200 ML blood/day. The treatment of the underlying destroyed lungs is usually radical surgery amounting to lobectomy or sometimes in severe cases, pneumonectomy. Many patients are not suitable candidates for radical surgery due to advanced age or associated co-morbid conditions. In these patients and in those in whom extensive resection of destroyed lung is not considered necessary, catheter based bronchial artery embolization (BAE) offers a safe and effective alternative therapy for cessation of hemoptysis. Its efficacy is heavily dependant on the experience of the operator. Certain safety precautions detailed in this chapter are necessary while performing BAE successfully and uneventfully. BAE also has much less morbidity than surgery and offers better quality of life compared to radical lobectomies and pneumonectomies.

Keywords Bronchial artery • Embolization • Hemoptysis • Pulmonary artery

Massive hemoptysis is a frightening and life-threatening condition. Treated conservatively the mortality may be upto 75 %, most often due to asphyxia [1, 2]. Massive hemoptysis has been variously defined as the expectoration of 100–600 ml of blood in 24–48 hours [1–3]. In developing countries, tuberculosis and post tubercular bronchiectasis account for the majority of patients presenting severe hemoptysis, but numerous other disease conditions may be associated with massive hemoptysis. These include cystic fibrosis, lung malignancy (including metastases), bronchiectasis, pneumonia, lung abscess, aspergilloma (isolated or associated with tuberculosis, sarcoid, etc), pneumoconiosis and pulmonary arteriovenous malformations. In many cases the bleeding arises from enlarged and tortuous bronchial arteries, but in several other cases, the source of bleeding is from enlarged collaterals from non-bronchial arteries. Rarely pseudo-aneurysms in the pulmonary artery branches may be responsible for the bleeding. Until a few years ago, surgery was considered the treatment of choice, but even in dedicated

© Springer International Publishing Switzerland 2017

K. Varghese, S. Adhyapak, *Therapeutic Embolization*,
DOI 10.1007/978-3-319-42494-1_3

respiratory centers, the surgical mortality is around 17 % and may be as high as 40 % when performed as an emergency [3, 4]. The first successful Bronchial Artery Embolization (BAE) for massive hemoptysis was reported by Remy et al [5]. Despite the well known risks of spinal trauma following BAE, several other reports have established that the procedure can be successfully performed provided the operator is aware of the potential complications and adequate precautions are taken. BAE is often the only option available for patients who are unsuitable for surgery due to significant comorbidities or poor respiratory reserve. BAE is minimally invasive, safe in experienced hands, effective in managementof hemoptysis and can be safely repeated in patients with recurrence of hemoptysis. Consequently, BAE is now an accepted and fairly widely performed procedure for the management of severe or recurrent hemoptysis.

The Clinical Significance of the Development of Pulmonary Collateral Circulation

The normal lung is supplied by two circulations of distinctly different origins, proportions, and functions. One is the pulmonary circulation which arises from the right heart, accounts for 99% of the arterial blood supply and delivers the systemic venous return to the lungs for gas exchange, while the second circulation consists of the bronchial arteries which are diminutive branches of the aorta delivering oxygenated blood to the lungs for the sustenance of its tissues, nerves, vessels, and conducting airways and constitute the remaining 1% of the arterial supply. Vascular connections between the two circulations are rare and if present, usually require elaborate injection techniques for their display as they are very diminutive and difficult to demonstrate.

In diseases which cause parenchymal fibrocavitatory changes, parenchymal destruction or chronic inflammation, the pulmonary circulation is compromised due to hypoxic vasoconstriction, thrombosis or vasculitis. In these conditions the systemic arteries supplying blood to the lung enlarge, become tortuous and hypertensive. Hypoxia and inflammatory processes result in the release of angiogenic growth factors due to which the pre-existing small vessels enlarge and become tortuous. New vessels appear, often recruited from adjacent systemic arteries and they join with the pre-existing arteries to form bizarre Medusan patterns (Fig. 3.1). The bronchial arteries and the new collateral vessels thus formed are usually thin walled but are subjected to systemic arterial pressure and could produce torrential bleeding should rupture occur. Patients with massive hemoptysis often die of asphyxia rather than exsanguination and it is estimated that about 400 ml of blood in the alveoli is sufficient to produce asphyxia [6]. In contrast to the normal lung, in which pre-capillary communications between the two circulations are difficult to demonstrate, the enlarged pre-capillary anastomoses between the pulmonary and systemic circulations are easily demonstrable in disease states.

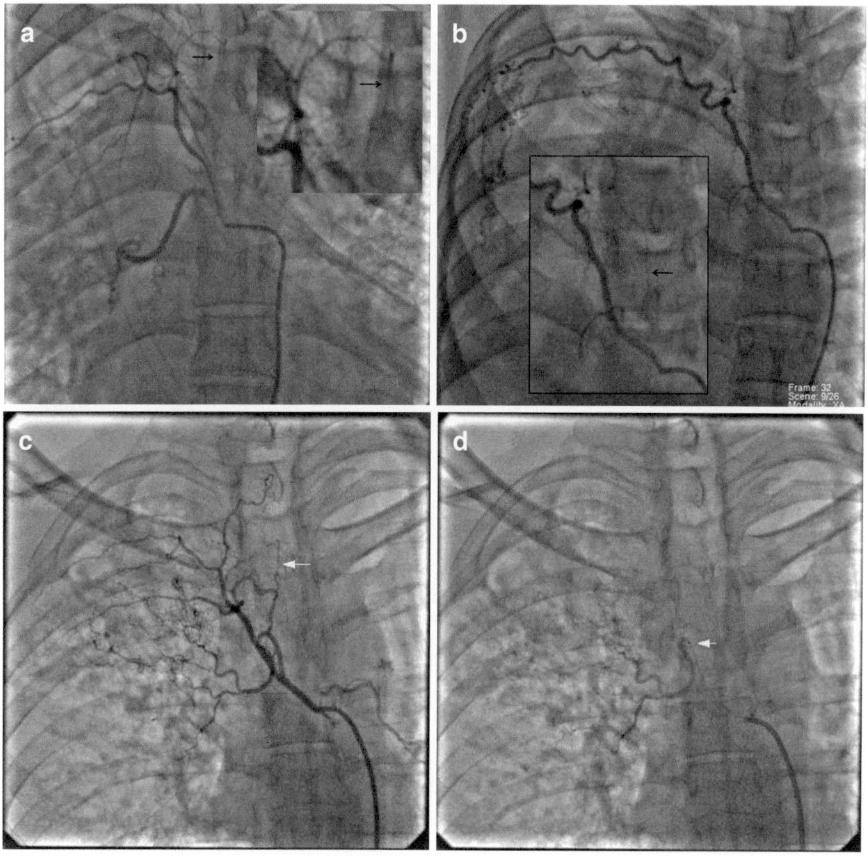

Fig. 3.1 (**a–c**) Spinal arteries arising from the thoracic aorta. Anterior medullary spinal arteries, the recognition of which are very essential in planning BAE. These tend to be parallel to the spine and remain in close proximity to the spine even in oblique views. Dorsal and ventral radicular arteries are small vessels arising from the segmental spinal arteries which supply the dorsal and ventral spinal roots (Inset). (**d**) Use of a microcatheter to cannulate the distal segments of the spinal artery from which the collaterals arise

Functions of the Pulmonary Collateral Circulation

In the normal lung, the collateral arterial circulation is too diminutive and serves only a nutrient function.

The hypertrophied collateral arterial circulation associated with localized pulmonary lesions does not have any appreciable hemodynamic effect on the pulmonary circulation, the left heart, or the systemic circulation. Although hypertrophied and hypertensive, they do not cause any significant hemodynamic effects although connecting the systemic circulation to the pulmonary circulation. They are not large enough to result in a significant left to right shunt.

The hypertrophied collateral circulation has been shown to affect the pulmonary circulation by diverting mixed venous blood away from diseased areas only in patients with extensive parenchymal lung disease. The increment in pulmonary blood flow contributed by the collateral arterial circulation may aggravate pulmonary hypertension in patients with diffuse restriction of the pulmonary vascular bed as in patients with significant loss of lung parenchyma and in patients with severe pulmonary hypertension.

Development of Hemoptysis

Different portions of the pulmonary collateral circulation may be responsible for hemoptysis in different diseases. In pulmonary disease, the arterial portion is responsible for hemoptysis. In mitral stenosis, the venous portion is responsible, and in pulmonary infarction, hemoptysis is due to an imbalance between the two collateral circulations [7]. The evaluation of a patient presenting with major hemoptysis should focus on determining the underlying pathology and the location of bleeding. While bronchoscopy is generally performed in such patients, evaluation if often difficult due to the presence of blood in the airways and it has <50 % accuracy in localizing the location of the bleeding. Chest Radiography is widely available and often gives valuable information regarding the underlying pathology especially in patients with active or healed tuberculosis. From an interventional viewpoint, it is useful to know the nature and location of the underlying pathology responsible for the hemoptysis. Contrast enhanced Computerised Tomography (CT) can localize the location of bleeding in 63–100 % of patients and has considerable value in diagnosing the underlying disease process. (Chun: see above). Both bronchial and non-bronchial arteries can be reliably identified as well as Rasmussen's aneurysms arising from the branches of the Pulmonary artery.

Anatomy of the Bronchial Arteries

Interventionalists who perform bronchial artery embolization (BAE) should have a thorough knowledge of bronchial artery anatomy. The bronchial arteries supply the trachea, extra- and intrapulmonary airways, bronchovascular bundles, nerves, supporting structures, regional lymph nodes, visceral pleura, and esophagus as well as the vasa vasora of the aorta, pulmonary artery, and pulmonary vein [33]. The bronchial arteries have variable anatomy in terms of origin, branching pattern, and course [8]. The bronchial arteries originate directly from the descending thoracic aorta, between the levels of the T5 and T6 vertebrae [9]. During angiography, we find that in the majority of patients, the bronchial artery (arteries) arises from the anterior aspect of the descending thoracic aorta at the level where the left main bronchus crosses the aorta and this constitutes a useful radiological landmark. Non bronchial arteries supplying abnormal collateral flow to diseased areas of the lung may arise from a variety of other locations. Cauldwell et al. [9] reported four classic bronchial artery branching patterns: two on the left and one on the right that presents as an intercostobronchial trunk (ICBT) in 40 % of cases; one on the left and one ICBT on the right in 21 % of cases; two on the left and two on the right (one ICBT and one bronchial artery) in 20 % of cases; and one on the left and two on the right (one ICBT and one bronchial artery) in 9.7 % of cases. The right ICBT is the most consistently seen vessel at angiography, seen in 80 % of individuals. The right ICBT usually arises from the right lateral aspect of the aorta while the left intercostal arteries arise from the posterior aspect of the aorta. After engaging the right intercostal artery, a slight anticlockwise rotation of the catheter causing the tip to point posteriorly and slightly to the left will usually result in the catheter engaging the ostium of the left intercostal artery. The other left intercostal arteries can then be selectively cannulated by moving the catheter up or down the aorta while maintaining the same orientation of the catheter.

Rarely bronchial arteries originate above T5 and below T6 vertebrae at the level of the major bronchi and are considered to be anomalous [9, 11]. The reported prevalence of bronchial arteries with an anomalous origin ranges from 8.3 to 35 % [11, 12]. Anomalous bronchial arteries may originate from the aortic arch, internal mammary artery, thyrocervical trunk, subclavian artery, costocervical trunk, brachiocephalic artery, pericardiacophrenic artery, inferior phrenic artery, or abdominal aorta. These anomalous bronchial arteries can be distinguished anatomically and angiographically from nonbronchial systemic collateral vessels in that they extend along the course of the major bronchi. In contrast, non-bronchial systemic collateral vessels enter the pulmonary parenchyma through the adherent pleura or via the pulmonary ligament, and a course which is not parallel to that of the bronchi [11]. The majority of anomalous bronchial arteries originate from the aortic arch [9, 11]. One should be aware of the possible presence of anomalous bronchial arteries, especially when a significant bronchial arterial supply to areas of abnormal pulmonary parenchyma is not demonstrated during a catheter search or descending thoracic aortography [13]. In addition, bronchial arteries of anomalous origin should be suspected and investigated angiographically in patients who present with recurrent hemoptysis despite successful embolization and in those in whom the source of bleeding has not been detected [11].

It is extremely important to be aware of the presence of spinal arteries while doing a bronchial artery embolization. Inadvertent embolization of spinal artery branches may result in disastrous neurological complications.

Two kinds of spinal arteries may be seen at bronchial and intercostal angiography during BAE. Dorsal and ventral radicular arteries (Fig. 3.1a–c) are small vessels that arise from segmental spinal arteries and supply the dorsal and ventral roots.

An average of eight anterior medullary arteries reinforce the anterior spinal artery, which is the major independent source of spinal cord perfusion. The artery of Adamkiewicz, or greater anterior medullary artery, reinforces the circulation of lumbar portion of the spinal cord. This unilateral vessel has been observed to arise between T9 and T12 in 75 % of cases [14]. The anterior medullary arteries often have a characteristic "hairpin" configuration at angiography. Radicular spinal arteries are often visualized during BAE. Anterior medullary arteries are rarely seen, but embolization in close proximity to them and repeat angiography of the collaterals near them should be avoided as spinal cord ischemia may occur with embolization. It has been suggested that rarely the spinal arteries may arise from the intercostal branch of the right ICBT in about 5–10 % of cases, but it is generally believed that their true prevalence is considerably lower [9]. The identification of spinal arteries is crucial during BAE. They are easily identified as vertical branches running parallel to the spinal column. When oblique views are visualized, spinal arteries continue to be visualized in close proximity to the spinal column. They do not move away from the spine in the oblique views.

CT Scan On CT scan, in adults, normal bronchial arteries measure less than 1.5 mm in diameter at their origin and 0.5 mm at their point of entry into a bronchopulmonary segment [17]. Therefore, a bronchial artery larger than 2 mm is most likely abnormal [18].

The hypertrophied bronchial arteries are visualized as enhancing nodular or tubular structures within the mediastinum or around the central airway on contrast-enhanced CT scans [47]. The primary locations of enlarged bronchial arteries are the retro-esophageal area, retro-tracheal area, retro-bronchial area, posterior wall of the main bronchus, and aorto-pulmonary window.

The common pitfalls include mis- diagnosing them with mediastinal lymph nodes, the azygos vein, and an enhancing esophageal wall which can all mimic the bronchial arteries on CT [19].

Agents Used for BAE

Embolic Agents

The most widely used embolic agents are polyvinyl alcohol particles of 350–500 mm and gelatin sponge pledgets or shavings. Polyvinyl alcohol particles are preferred to gelatin sponge pledgets because the pledgets are resorbable and may not provide as durable a result and cause recanalization resulting in recurrence of hemoptysis [20]. An experimental study has demonstrated a bronchopulmonary anastomosis with a diameter of 325 μm in the human lung. Therefore, it has been inferred that pulmonary infarction via bronchial artery–pulmonary artery shunts or systemic artery embolization via bronchial artery– pulmonary vein shunts may occur when embolic agents less than 325 μm in diameter are used. In addition, it is important to avoid using embolic agents that produce distal occlusion to such an extent that normal peripheral branches that supply the bronchi, esophagus, or vasa vasorum of the pulmonary artery or aorta become occluded. Hence, PVA particles of 300–500 μm have been found to be ideal for BAE. Microspheres have also been reportedly used as successful embolization material [21].

To avoid non-target damage to small normal collaterals and the risk of necrosis to surrounding structures such as the aortic, esophageal, bronchial, or pulmonary artery walls, smaller particles or liquid embolic agents should be avoided [22]. Coils

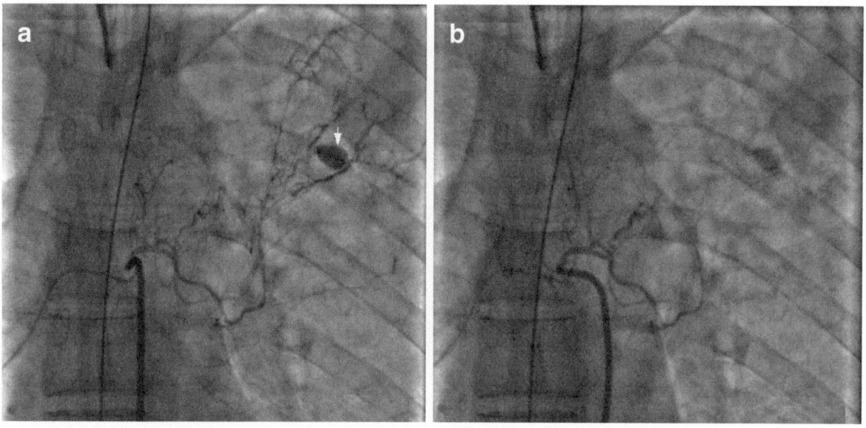

Fig. 3.2 (**a**) Rasmussen's aneurysm seen in the bronchial angiogram (*highlighted by white arrow*) and (**b**) Rasmussen's aneurysm after embolization. Image provided courtesy of Boston Scientific. © 2014 Boston Scientific Corporation or its affiliates. All rights reserved

should be avoided to preserve access to future sites of bronchial bleeding and allow retreatment of an affected vessel [22]. The placement of coils in the proximal portion of the collaterals limits future embolizations to progressively smaller and less accessible collateral vessels distal to them. Coils may, however, have a role in the treatment of arterial aneurysms called Rasmussen's aneurysms or pseudoaneurysms or in therapeutic occlusion of an internal mammary artery to protect surrounding normal territory and avoid backfilling via collaterals (Fig. 3.2a, b).

Contraindications for BAE

The only real contraindications for bronchial artery embolization (BAE) are the usual contraindications, absolute or relative, for angiography in general including uncorrectable coagulopathy, renal failure, and severe contrast allergy. Since BAE is often needed as a lifesaving procedure, the risk benefit ratio often favors performance of the procedure.

Preprocedure Evaluation and Work-Up

Preprocedure workup is performed with the goal of determining the cause of the hemoptysis and to guide location of endovascular therapy [22]. Other sources of hemoptysis from the nasopharynx, gastrointestinal tract, or oropharynx should be excluded [23]. Angiographic localization of the origin of the abnormal vessels can assist in a prompt, directed, and efficient procedure, with decreased procedure time.

Radiography, bronchoscopy, CT, and CT angiography have all been used for pre operative localization. Conventional chest radiography is a quick, noninvasive, and widely available first step that can localize the site of abnormality in 19–83 % of cases [22].

Traditionally, bronchoscopy was considered an important step before embolization, with the expectation that the site could be easily localized, leading to more rapid and specifically directed embolization.

The reported success of bronchoscopy in lateralizing the side of bleeding is 49–93 % [22]. However, in the setting of a normal radiograph bronchoscopy only adds additional localizing information in 0–31 % of cases [22]. More recent reports suggest that bronchoscopy may be less useful than thought, due to poor localization of bleeding in the setting of massive hemoptysis with little added benefit if location and etiology of bleeding is known radiographically [12, 24–26].

Computed tomography and CT angiography can localize the site of bleeding in 63–100 % of cases [25, 27]. Specifically, CT can aid in diagnosing non-bronchial systemic supply in 80 % of cases.

A variety of opinions exist regarding whether pre-embolization CT or bronchoscopy should be performed, with the final decision in each case requiring balancing the possibility of improved pre-procedure information against possible delay in definitive treatment, especially in the setting of a life threatening condition. A practical approach may be CT angiography in a non-acute setting, with the goals of identifying the site and etiology of bleeding and determining the relevant anatomy, especially localization of the artery of Adamkiewicz [28]. In the setting of hemodynamic instability or acute airway compromise, the best approach would likely be chest radiograph followed directly by angiography with embolization.

Bronchial Artery Embolization

Angiographic Diagnosis

Angiographic findings indicating embolization of the affected vessel include: hypervascularity (83 %), tortuosity and enlarged bronchial arteries (31 %), shunting into pulmonary artery or vein (28 %), parenchymal staining (15 %), vascular abnormalities such as aneurysms (13 %), and extravasation into the airway (2–10.7 %) [29–31]. Visualization of bronchial arteries larger than 2–2.5 mm in diameter are considered enlarged and hypertrophied [22].

Technique

There are two differing techniques for BAE. In patients presenting with the first episode of hemoptysis, initially a descending thoracic aortogram is done to demonstrate the enlarged bronchial arteries. If there are no bronchial arteries visualized, selective cannulation and angiography of systemic vessels; subclavian arteries, internal mammary arteries, intercostals arteries, thyrocervical trunk, costocervical trunk and in the case of lower lobe disease, inferior phrenic artery is performed. In patients presenting with recurrence of hemoptysis, non-bronchial artery angiograms should be performed as a rule (Figs. 3.3, 3.4a, b, 3.5a, b, 3.6a, b, 3.7a, b, 3.8a, b, 3.9a, b, 3.10a, b, 3.11a, b and 3.12a, b). An alternative technique would be to begin the procedure with a diagnostic aortography to visualize large/abnormal bronchopulmonary collateral arteries.

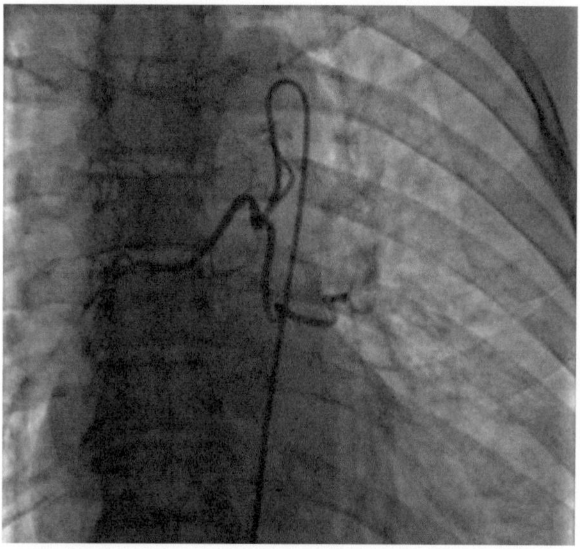

Fig. 3.3 Use of a reverse *curve* catheter to cannulate the bronchopulmonary collaterals and embolize them

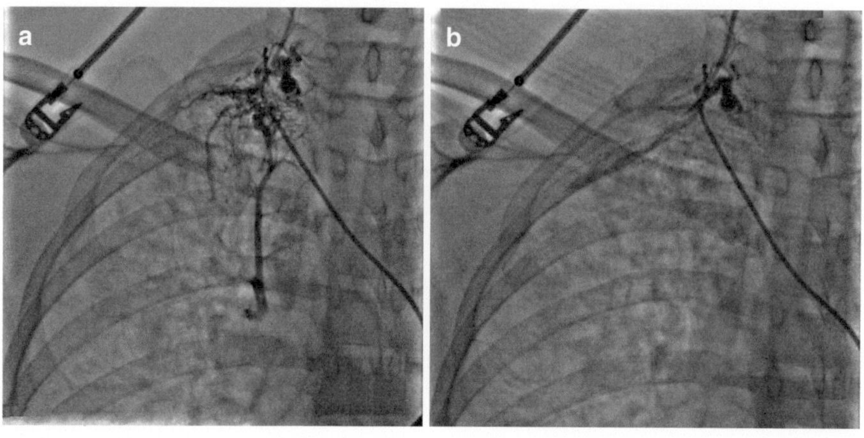

Fig. 3.4 Collaterals connecting the costocervical trunk and a branch of the pulmonary artery, (**a**) before embolization and (**b**) after embolization

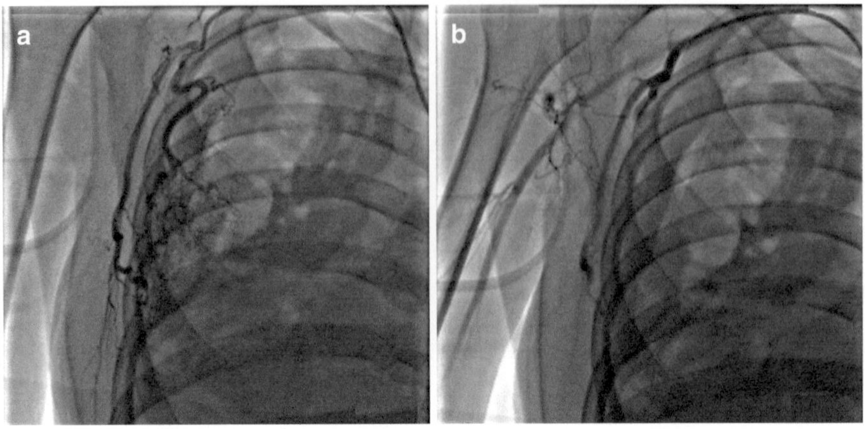

Fig. 3.5 Collaterals arising from the Axillary artery, before embolisation (**a**) and after embolization (**b**)

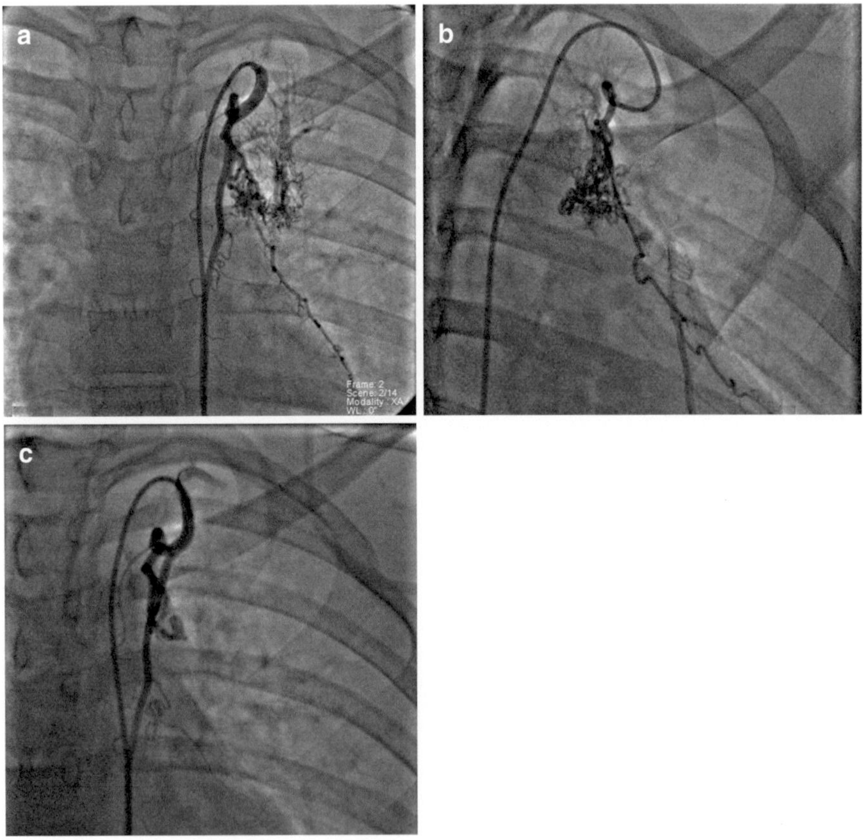

Fig. 3.6 (**a–c**) Collaterals connecting LIMA (Left Internal Mammary Artery) and the pulmonary circulation before embolization. (**b**) shows selective cannulation of the feeding branch arising from LIMA and (**c**) disappearance of collaterals after embolization

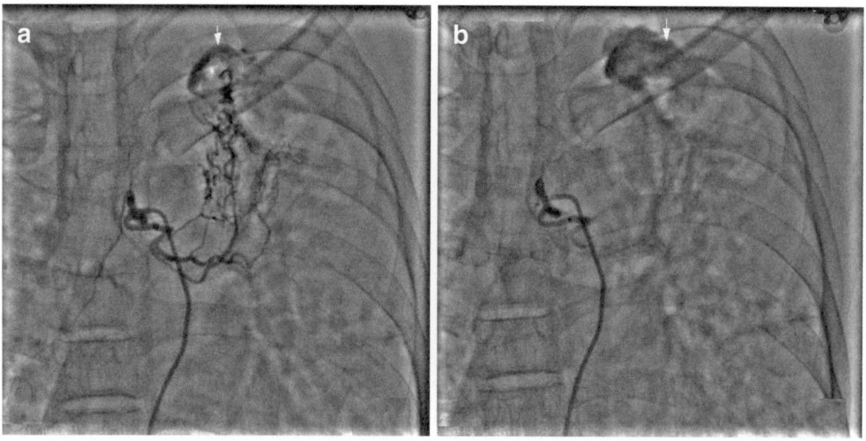

Fig. 3.7 (**a**, **b**) Collaterals from left bronchial artery with extravasation of contrast into the lung parenchyma (*white arrow*) signifying active bleed and (**b**) obliteration of collaterals post embolization

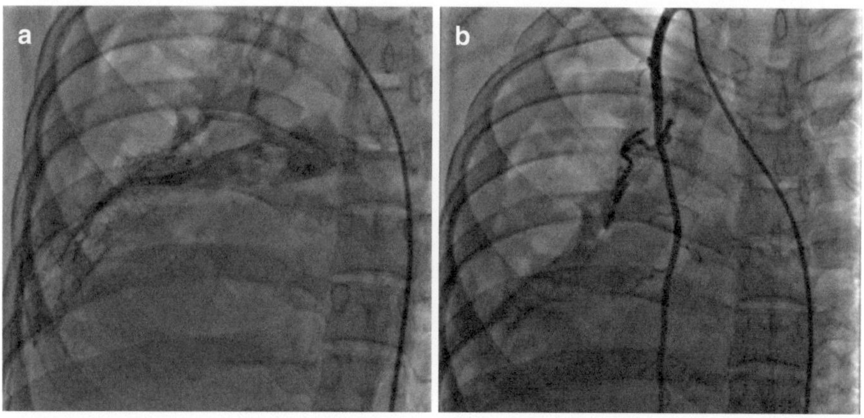

Fig. 3.8 (**a**, **b**) Collaterals from the Right internal mammary artery (RIMA) seen draining into the pulmonary vein (**a**), and post embolization (**b**) occlusion of collaterals

Before embolization, high-quality diagnostic bronchial angiograms should be performed and carefully examined for presence of the any spinal artery branches to avoid inadvertent embolization. If findings are equivocal, an oblique view may be useful. The spinal arteries course along the spine even when visualized in the oblique views.

If any spinal artery branches are seen arising from an affected bronchial artery, extreme precaution should be taken to avoid potentially catastrophic neurological complications. Frequent check angiograms should be performed during an embolization procedure even when spinal branches are not visualized during the initial angiogram. Due to the brisk flow into the broncho-pulmonary collaterals, spinal

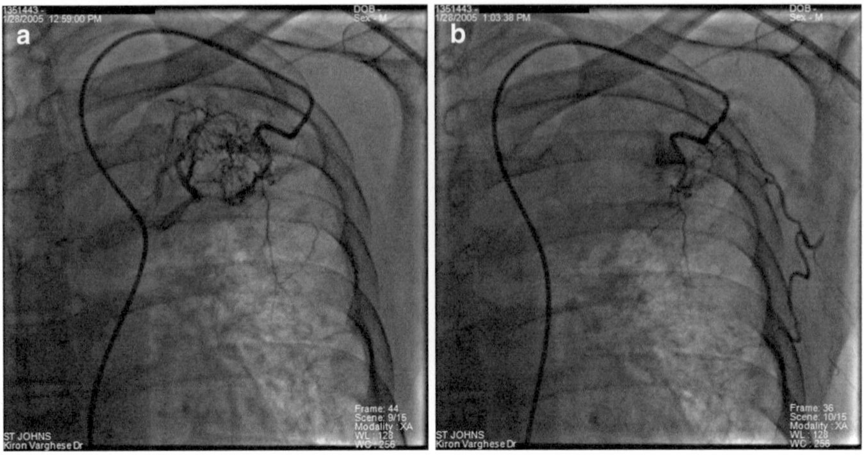

Fig. 3.9 (**a**, **b**) Collaterals from the thoraco acromial artery to the pulmonary circulation, before embolisation. (**a**) and after embolization (**b**)

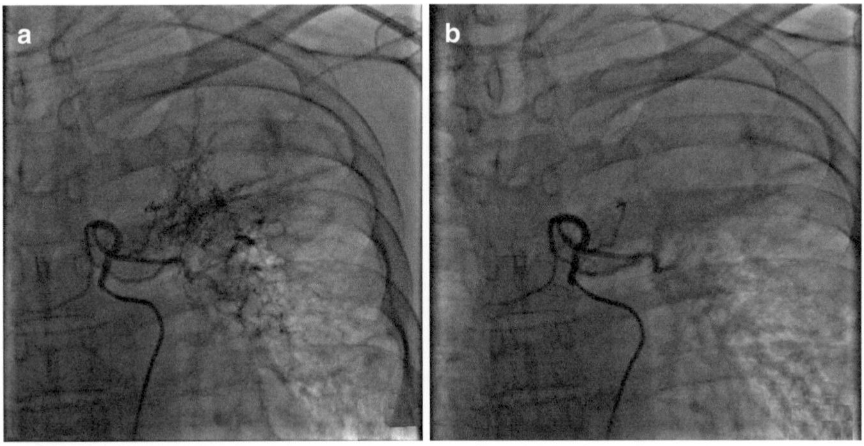

Fig. 3.10 (**a**) Angiogram showing common origin of left and right bronchial arteries with hypervascularity and enlargement of the left bronchial artery and (**b**) disappearance of collaterals following embolization. Note the sharp upward origin of the bronchial artery which is easily cannulated using an Amplatz coronary catheter or a reverse curve catheter (eg Simmons catheter) without forming the reverse loop

branches and communications with other arteries are often visualized only after partial embolization is performed [30–32]. The following measures will help to reduce the risk of spinal ischemia:

1. Suitable catheters should be chosen to provide stable support without significant damping of pressure.
2. A microcatheter can be positioned beyond the origin of the spinal branch and embolization performed via the microcatheter.

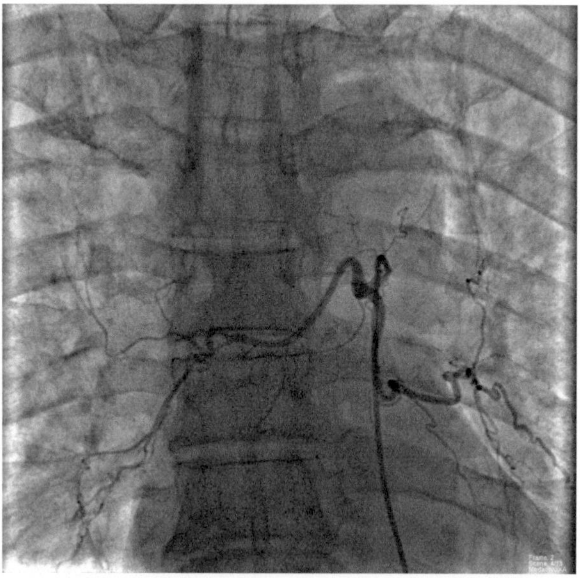

Fig. 3.11 Bronchial angiogram demonstrating the common origin of two bronchial arteries from the thoracic aorta

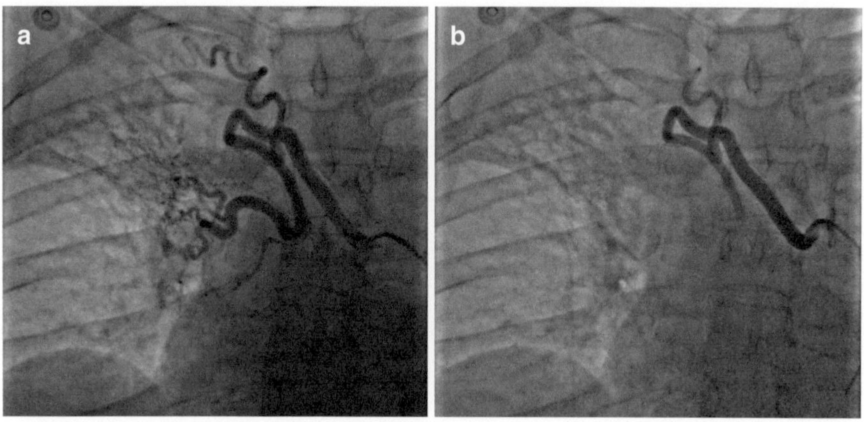

Fig. 3.12 (a, b) Bronchial angiogram demonstrating the hypertrophied tortuous transformation of the bronchial artery due to increased flow and embolisation of collaterals arising from them to the pulmonary circulation

3. Care should be taken to inject slowly and avoid reflux of embolic material and hence embolization should be stopped when flow becomes sluggish.
4. Larger size particles (eg: 500 micron) are less likely to traverse into the spinal branches and may be safer.
5. It is prudent to perform all embolisations under fluoroscopy, do check angiograms when flow becomes sluggish and also to check frequently for damping of pressure.

6. Many patients have multiple arteries supplying bronchopulmonary collaterals and when faced with a challenging anatomy, opting not to embolise an artery which also supplies spinal artery branches may be a wise decision.

A variety of 4 F or 5 F curved tip catheters like Cobra, Renal double curve, Right Amplatz or Judkins Right coronary catheters can be used for delineation of the bronchial arteries (Fig. 3.3). Reverse curve catheters eg SOS catheter, may be necessary for arteries with an inferiorly oriented origin. The tip is placed at the top of the descending thoracic aorta and directed to the right or posterolaterally to search for the right ICBT and left posterolaterally to search for left bronchials [10, 20]. Hand injections of 2 to 7 cc of contrast can be performed for each selected bronchial vessel. If abnormal findings are present, embolizations can be performed, the object being to embolize the distal bed. Another safety precaution to be followed is after stable catheter placement, embolization should be done under continuous fluoroscopic visualization until flow in the embolized vessel is significantly slow. At that point, the remaining embolic material is flushed with saline and check angiography performed with the goal of achieving distal stasis in the vessel while avoiding reflux back into normal circulation. Proximal occlusion (e.g. coil embolization) should be carefully avoided in order to permit future embolizations of the distal bed, in case of recurrence of hemoptysis. [10]. The descending thoracic aorta should be evaluated between T4 and T8 levels. Embolization of all visualized abnormal bronchial arteries should be performed. The use of a 3 F microcatheter helps in superselective embolization of smaller distal collaterals and prevents complications especially when spinal artery branches are seen to srise from them (Fig. 3.1d).

Intercostal angiograms are required to delineate systemic collaterals arising from them. The right intercostals arteries usually arise laterally (Fig. 3.13a, b), whereas the left intercostals arteries arise posterolaterally from the thoracic aorta (Fig. 3.14a, b). Bilateral subclavian angiography must be performed, especially in

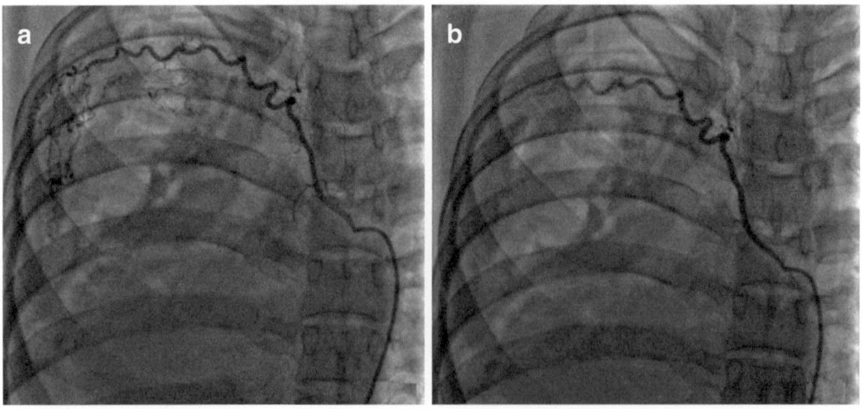

Fig. 3.13 Angiogram demonstrating the origin of the right intercostals artery from the lateral aspect of the thoracic aorta (**a**) and disappearance of the collaterals post embolization (**b**)

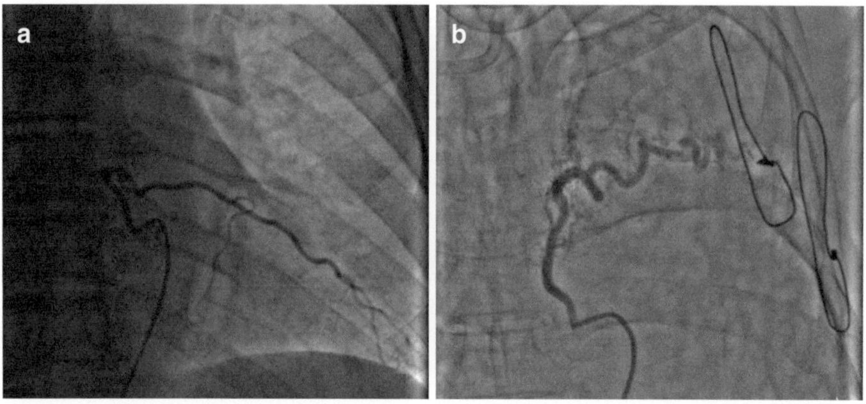

Fig. 3.14 (**a**, **b**) Angiograms of the left intercostals artery of two patients demonstrating the posterolateral origin from the thoracic aorta

the patients with recurrence of hemoptysis. A thoracic aortogram may also be indicated in these situations for visualization of the non-bronchial systemic collaterals. If lower lobe origin is suspected, a lower thoracic/upper abdominal aortogram may help determine the phrenic artery source [10]. If no bronchial arterial or systemic arterial source is found, a pulmonary angiogram should be performed to exclude entities such as pulmonary artery aneurysms, arteriovenous malformations and fistulas [20].

Clinical Outcomes

The technical success rates of embolization range from 65 to 100 % [29, 34]. More recent reports have had higher technical success rates of 90–94 %, likely due to increased use of superselective techniques and increased use of permanent, rather than absorbable, embolization materials [21, 35, 36]. Recurrent bleeding can be seen in 10–50 % of patients [22]. The short-term bleeding recurrence rate, within 1 month, is reported to be from 10 to 49 %. Greater than 30-day recurrence rates range between 10 and 52 % [37–40]. The causes for recurrent bleeding include; progression of underlying disease, recanalization or revascularization, incomplete embolization, and emergence of other vascular supply to the affected area, such as from systemic collaterals [22]. The recurrence rates depend on the underlying etiology of the lung disease, being higher in the setting of infections such as chronic tuberculosis (15.5 %), with aspergilloma (75 %), and in neoplasms (42 %) and lesser in bronchiectasis [22, 38, 40]. In one series of 18 patients with cystic fibrosis, hemoptysis was controlled with the first embolization in 75 %, after the second session in 89 %, and after the third in 93 % of patients. In this series, the chances of the source of bleeding arising from non-bronchial systemic collaterals was 75 % in patients who had recurrent bleeding versus 8 % in those being treated for the first time. This is likely to represent successful embolization of the bronchial artery supply, with later recruitment of systemic collaterals due to an underlying chronic disease.

Complications of BAE

The complication rates associated with BAE have reduced with improvisations in technique attributable to the use of microcatheters for superselective embolization and use of permanent embolizing materials.

Rarely, paraplegia, transient paraparesis, and transient Brown-Se'quard syndrome have been reported following bronchial artery embolizations, with an overall risk of transverse myelitis less than 1 % [36, 37, 41]. Postembolization syndrome, consisting of retrosternal chest pain, intercostal pain, transient dysphagia, and fever is not uncommon [20]. Other reported complications include stroke, esophageal ulceration, bronchial infarction and stenosis, bronchoesophageal fistula, transient left orbital and forehead pain, and transient neurological symptoms [22, 36–38]. As spinal cord branches are often not visualized until after embolization, suggesting that they are often small, super selective microcatheter techniques are associated with lower risk of complications in these situations [32–34, 42].

In some anecdotal reports, transient blindness has been reported following BAE due to cortical blindness [43]. CT scans have been normal with no evidence of ischemic infarcts. There was no central retinal artery occlusion on fundal examination. It has been hypothesized that the cortical blindness develops because of embolism of the particles to the occipital cortex in both hemispheres, either through a bronchial artery to pulmonary vein connection or through collaterals between the bronchial and vertebral arteries. This complication has been strongly associated with use of liquid embolic agents and smaller particles. Embolic agents, such as gelfoam, absolute alcohol, ivalon, and isobutyl-2-cyanoarcylate have been reported to cause ischaemic complication in adjacent structures. These liquid agents or small particles can cause tissue infarction of adjacent structures due to distal vascular occlusion. When right to left shunting is present, these liquid agents or small particles can also embolize into the systemic circulation to cause distant structure ischaemia. Therefore, embolic particles should be at least 200–300 μm in size and larger (300–500 μm) when shunting is identified on the diagnostic angiogram.

Our Experience with BAE

Between January 2002 and April 2014, 148 patients, 116 males and 32 females aged 18–65 years with massive hemoptysis were subjected to BAE. Selective cannulation of the descending thoracic aortic branches was performed. The catheters used were 5 F and 6 F right Judkin's, Reuter, Renal double curve and Cobra C2 catheters. All collaterals were embolised using 200–1000 μm poly vinyl alcohol particles.

The etiology of hemoptysis in majority of our patients was tuberculosis (74.5 % n = 110). Bronchiectasis not related to tuberculosis was seen in 11.5 % [23]. Aspergilloma in 6.1 % [16] patients and was idiopathic in the rest. Mean follow up period was 27 months.

Embolisation succeeded in cessation of hemoptysis immediately after the procedure in 95.3 % of patients. There was no procedure related mortality. One patient developed transient monoparesis which recovered in one day and another patient who underwent BAE of multiple vessels on multiple occasions due to recurrence of hemoptysis developed transient urinary retention possibly due to bladder paresis. Transient chest pain was a common complaint especially with the use of ionic contrast media with a few patients continuing to have minor chest pain for a few hours. Three patients complained of pain in the eyes but had no visual loss. One patient with massive hemoptysis and multiple bronchopulmonary collaterals developed contrast induced nephropathy which resolved completely. Five patients were intubated and on ventilator support at the time of BAE. In hospital mortality was seen in 2.8 % [11] patients, one due to recurrent hemoptysis and the remaining due to respiratory complications. Recurrence of hemoptysis requiring re embolisation was seen in 20.9 %. These were due to re-canalization of the embolized vessels or formation of new vessels in patients with underlying chronic tuberculosis.

Conclusions

Acute massive hemoptysis or chronic recurrent hemoptysis are potentially life-threatening conditions, with the majority caused by hypertrophied bronchial arteries in response to a pulmonary parenchymal abnormality. Bronchial artery embolization is a well-established treatment with an excellent short-term success rate and an acceptable long-term success rate in what are often chronic diseases with limited surgical options. When performed by an experienced operator with appropriate precautions, it is safe and well-tolerated with favorable clinical outcomes and acceptable procedural complication rate.

References

1. Crocco JA, Rooney JJ, Fankushen DS et al. Massivehaemoptysis. Arch Intern Med. 1968; 121:495.
2. Chun J, Morgan R. Cardiovasc Intervent Radiol. 2010;33:240–250.
3. Fernando et al. Cardiovasc Intervent Radiol. 2010;33:240–250.
4. Marshal TJ and Jackson JE: Cardiovasc Intervent Radiol. 2010;33:240–250.
5. Remy J, Voisin C, Dupuis C et al. Traitement des hemoptysies par embolization de la circulation systemique. Ann Radiol (Paris). 1974;17:5.
6. Jean-Baptiste E. Clinical assessment and management of massive hemoptysis. Crit Care Med. 2000;28:1642–1647.
7. Fishman AP. The clinical significance of the pulmonary collateral circulation. Circulation. 1961;24:677–90.

8. Lippert H, Pabst R. Bronchial arteries. In: Lippert H, Pabst R, editors. Arterial variations in man. Munich: Bergmann Verlag; 1985. p. 18–9.
9. Cauldwell EW, Siekert RG, Lininger RE, Anson BJ. The bronchial arteries: an anatomic study of 105 human cadavers. Surg Gynecol Obstet. 1948;86:395–412.
10. Stoll JF, Bettmann MA. Bronchial artery embolization to control hemoptysis: a review. Cardiovasc Intervent Radiol. 1988;11(5):263–9.
11. Sancho C, Escalante E, Dominguez J, et al. Embolization of bronchial arteries of anomalous origin. Cardiovasc Intervent Radiol. 1998;21:300–4.
12. Cohen AM, Doershuk CF, Stern RC. Bronchial artery embolization to control hemoptysis in cystic fibrosis. Radiology. 1990;175:401–5.
13. McPherson S, Routh WD, Nath H, Keller FS. Anomalous origin of bronchial arteries: potential pitfall of embolotherapy for hemoptysis. J Vasc Interv Radiol. 1990;1:86–8.
14. Rosenthal D. Spinal cord ischemia after abdominal aortic operation: is it preventable? J Vasc Surg. 1999;30:391–9.
15. Uflacker R, Kaemmerer A, Neves C, Picon PD. Management of massive hemoptysis by bronchial artery embolization. Radiology. 1983;146:627–34.
16. Uflacker R, Kaemmerer A, Picon PD, et al. Bronchial artery embolization in the management of hemoptysis: technical aspects and long-term results. Radiology. 1985;157:637–44.
17. Deffenbach ME, Charan NB, Lakshminarayan S, Butler J. The bronchial circulation: small, but a vital attribute to the lung. Am Rev Respir Dis. 1987;135:463–81.
18. Furuse M, Saito K, Kunieda E, et al. Bronchial arteries: CT demonstration with arteriographic correlation. Radiology. 1987;162:393–8.
19. Song JW, Im JG, Shim YS, Park JH, Yeon KM, Han MC. Hypertrophied bronchial artery at thin-section CT in patients with bronchiectasis: correlation with CT angiographic findings. Radiology. 1998;208:187–91.
20. Roberts AC. Bronchial artery embolization therapy. J Thorac Imaging. 1990;5(4):60–72.
21. Corr PD. Bronchial artery embolization for life-threatening hemoptysis using tris-acryl microspheres: shortterm result. Cardiovasc Intervent Radiol. 2005;28(4):439–41.
22. Yoon W, Kim J, Kim Y, Chung T, Kang H. Bronchial and nonbronchial systemic artery embolization for life-threatening hemoptysis: a comprehensive review. Radiographics. 2002;22(6): 1395–409.
23. Thompson AB, Teschler H, Rennard SI. Pathogenesis, evaluation, and therapy for massive hemoptysis. Clin Chest Med. 1992;13(1):69–82.
24. Brinson GM, Noone PG, Mauro MA, et al. Bronchial artery embolization for the treatment of hemoptysis in patients with cystic fibrosis. Am J Respir Crit Care Med. 1998;157(6 Pt 1): 1951–8.
25. Hsiao EI, Kirsch CM, Kagawa FT, et al. Utility of fiberoptic bronchoscopy before bronchial artery embolization for massive hemoptysis. AJR Am J Roentgenol. 2001;177(4):861–7.
26. Sweezey NB, Fellows KE. Bronchial artery embolization for severe hemoptysis in cystic fibrosis. Chest. 1990;97(6):1322–6.
27. Abal AT, Nair PC, Cherian J. Haemoptysis: aetiology, evaluation and outcome–a prospective study in a third-world country. Respir Med. 2001;95(7):548–52.
28. Takase K, Sawamura Y, Igarashi K, et al. Demonstration of the artery of Adamkiewicz at multidetector row helical CT. Radiology. 2002;223(1):39–45.
29. Swanson KL, Johnson CM, Prakash UB, et al. Bronchial artery embolization: experience with 54 patients. Chest. 2002;121(3):789–95.
30. Re'my-Jardin M, Bouaziz N, Dumont P, et al. Bronchial and nonbronchial systemic arteries at multi-detector row CT angiography: comparison with conventional angiography. Radiology. 2004;233(3):741–9.
31. Ramakantan R, Bandekar V, Gandhi M, Aulakh B, Deshmukh H. Massive hemoptysis due to pulmonary tuberculosis: control with bronchial artery embolization. Radiology. 1996;200(3): 691–4.
32. White RI. Bronchial artery embolotherapy for control of acute hemoptysis: analysis of outcome. Chest. 1999;115(4):912–5.

33. Najarian KE, Morris CS. Arterial embolization in the chest. J Thorac Imaging. 1998; 13(2):93–104.
34. Andersen PE. Imaging and interventional radiological treatment of hemoptysis. Acta Radiol. 2006;47(8):780–92.
35. Marshall TJ, Jackson JE. Vascular intervention in the thorax: bronchial artery embolization for haemoptysis. Eur Radiol. 1997;7(8):1221–7.
36. Karmy-Jones R, Hastreiter D, Burdick T. Hemothorax complicating bronchial artery aneurysm. Can Respir J. 2005;12(5):279–81.
37. Bredin CP, Richardson PR, King TK, et al. Treatment of massive hemoptysis by combined occlusion of pulmonary and bronchial arteries. Am Rev Respir Dis. 1978;117(5):969–73.
38. Kato A, Kudo S, Matsumoto K, et al. Bronchial artery embolization for hemoptysis due to benign diseases: immediate and long-term results. Cardiovasc Intervent Radiol. 2000;23(5): 351–7.
39. Yu-Tang Goh P, Lin M, Teo N, En Shen Wong D. Embolization for hemoptysis: a six -year review. Cardiovasc Intervent Radiol. 2002;25(1):17–25.
40. Hayakawa K, Tanaka F, Torizuka T, et al. Bronchial artery embolization for hemoptysis: immediate and long-term results. Cardiovasc Intervent Radiol. 1992;15(3):154–8; discussion 158–159.
41. Mal H, Rullon I, Mellot F, et al. Immediate and long-term results of bronchial artery embolization for life-threatening hemoptysis. Chest. 1999;115(4):996–1001.
42. Tanaka N, Yamakado K, Murashima S, et al. Superselective bronchial artery embolization for hemoptysis with a coaxial microcatheter system. J Vasc Interv Radiol. 1997;8(1 Pt 1):65–70.
43. Liu SF, Lee TU, Wong SL, Lai YF, Lin AS. Transient cortical blindness: a complication of bronchial artery embolization. J Case Rep. 1997;4:983–6.

Chapter 4
Renal Artery Embolization for Bleeding, Angiolipoma, Renal Cell Carcinoma and Certain Medical Conditions

Abstract Renal artery embolization (RAE) is an effective minimally invasive alternative procedure for the treatment of a variety of surgical and chronic medical renal diseases. It is invaluable in containing bleeding due to iatrogenic and other traumatic causes which otherwise requires nephrectomy. Since the 1970s when RAE was first developed, technical advances and growing experience have expanded the indications to not only include treatment of conditions such as symptomatic hematuria and palliation for metastatic renal cancer, but also preoperative infarction of renal tumors, treatment of angiomyolipomas, vascular malformations, medical renal disease and complications following renal transplantation and biopsy. The availability of more precise embolic agents and smaller delivery catheters, have contributed to the growth of RAE for an exxpanding list of urologic and nephrologic conditions.

Keywords Renal artery • Embolization • Coils • Angiolipoma • Carcinoma

Introduction

Renal artery embolization is an effective minimally invasive alternative to surgery for the treatment, palliation, and prevention of a variety of conditions. Technical advances and increasing experience with renal artery embolization have expanded the range of its applications.

Vascular Anatomy

Knowledge of the classic anatomy and variations of the renal vessels is important in the planning prior to renal artery embolization. Careful evaluation for variant anatomy on preprocedural imaging using ultrasound, computed tomography (CT), or magnetic resonance imaging (MRI) would be helpful prior to RAE.

© Springer International Publishing Switzerland 2017
K. Varghese, S. Adhyapak, *Therapeutic Embolization*,
DOI 10.1007/978-3-319-42494-1_4

Classic Anatomy

The renal arteries arise from the anterolateral aspect of the abdominal aorta, below the origins of the coeliac trunk and the superior mesenteric artery, at the level of the L1–L2 intervertebral disc. Although the exact location may vary, 98 % of the main renal arteries and 74 % of the accessory renal arteries arise at a level between the upper margin of L1 and lower margin of L2 vertebrae. A single renal artery to both kidneys is found in 76 % of patients (Ozkan et al). Near the hilum of the kidney, each renal artery divides into an anterior and a posterior branch, which in turn, divide into upper, middle, and lower pole segmental arteries (Fig. 4.1). These segmental vessels bifurcate into lobar arteries, which then penetrate the renal parenchyma and divide into the interlobar arteries.

Variant Anatomy

With the gradual increase in renal interventions, knowledge of the anatomical variations in the renal arteries has attained greater importance and is often crucial to achieve the intended goals for various indications. There are two types of variant renal arteries.

The first variant is referred to as early division and is characterized by branching of the main renal arteries into segmental branches proximal to the hilum. The second variation is, known as the extra renal arteries which can be further divided into accessory (hilar) and aberrant (polar) arteries. Accessory renal arteries enter the hilum along with the main renal artery, while the aberrant renal arteries enter outside the hilum, directly through the capsule.

Upto 30 % of patients may have extra renal arteries which constitute the most common, clinically important vascular variation. Multiple renal arteries are unilateral in 24 % of patients and bilateral in 5–10 %. These extra renal arteries may arise from the aorta or iliac arteries at a level as high as the T11 vertebra down to the level of the L4 vertebra. Rarely, these arteries can take origin from the celiac artery, superior and inferior mesenteric arteries, middle colic artery, middle sacral artery or the lumbar arteries. In addition, there are reported cases of renal arteries arising from a common trunk and from the contralateral renal artery. Embryologically, this wide variation in anatomy can be explained by the incomplete involution of the mesonephric arteries, which form a network of arteries during development.

Accessory renal arteries, when present, enter the renal hilum and may perfuse the upper or lower renal poles (Fig. 4.2a–c). Most commonly, the accessory artery perfuses the lower pole and may be of clinical importance as it may cause obstruction by passing anterior to the uretero pelvic junction. A less common variant is a superior pole artery which arises from the aorta to supply a minor part of the upper renal pole. This artery is often so small that it may not be seen angiographically, but is seen on CT scan.

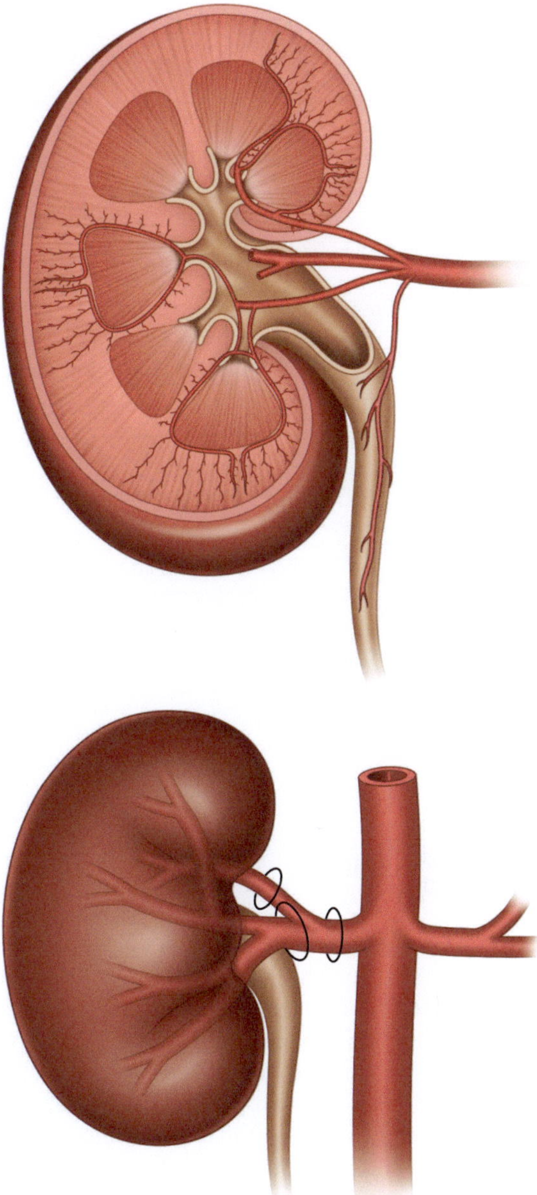

Fig. 4.1 The normal or classic renal artery anatomy

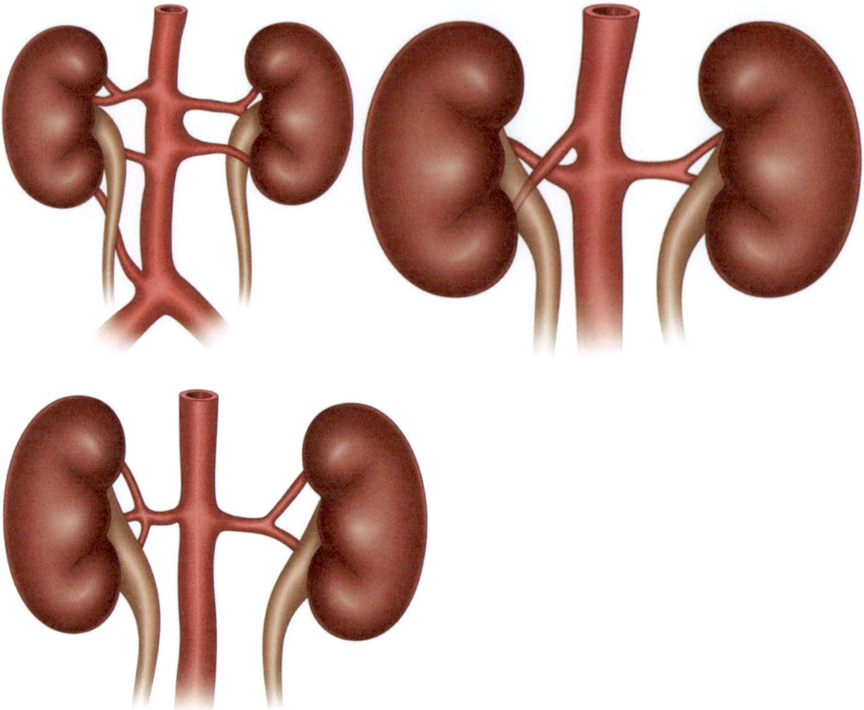

Fig. 4.2 (**a–c**) Normal variants in renal artery anatomy

Technical Details

Before the procedure, prophylactic antibiotic coverage is recommended in some centres, but we usually administer it only for diabetic or immunocompromised patients with an anticipated large area of necrosis. The procedure can be performed with local anesthesia to the access site and mild or no sedation, although some authors prefer general anesthesia [1]. Recommendations for general anesthesia may include cases in whom use of absolute alcohol is being considered as an embolic/sclerosing agent, particularly if large volumes (>10 mL) are being used. This is partly because of the procedure related pain and, more importantly, the small risk of cardiopulmonary collapse that may occur if large volumes of absolute alcohol reflux into the systemic circulation from the renal artery.

The ipsilateral or contralateral common femoral artery is commonly used for vascular access, although the brachial or radial artery is being increasingly used especially in patients with occluded femoral arteries. The left radial artery is preferred over the right radial artery due to the shorter distance to the renal artery. The upper limb approach may be more appropriate for interventions on renal arteries with a sharp downward angulation. The normal orientation of the renal arteries is horizontal, slightly posterior and caudal.

A variety of catheters have been used for catheterization of the main renal artery and its large branches, including a Cobra configured (C2) catheter, the Judkins Right coronary catheter, the RC-2 catheter and the Lev-1 catheter, reverse-angled catheters like the Simons catheters (Simons-1 and -2) and the SOS Omni catheter may be needed in some cases, especially for renal arteries with a downward origin. Engaging the renal artery may occasionally be difficult due to atherosclerotic disease of the aorta, abdominal aortic aneurysm, tortuosity or stenosis of the iliac arteries, narrowing of the renal artery orifice, or upward angulation of therenal arteries. Upward angled arteries can be due to large mass effect of renal cell carcinoma or an angiolipoma. Sometimes, a large hematoma can also cause a mass effect leading to distortion of renal arterial anatomy.

Specific parameters to consider for catheter selection include the diameter of the aorta at the level of the renal arteries, length of the main renal artery and its angle with respect to the axis of the aorta. The chance of successful embolization is optimized by ensuring that the catheter conforms to the vessel anatomy, particularly for small arteries. To achieve this, catheter exchanges over a wire may sometimes be needed [3]. Generally, small vessels can be approached via non-tapered 4F or 5F catheters alone or in combination with coaxial systems. Superselective catheterization of renal artery branches is often possible with 4 or 5F catheters, but may require the use of microcatheters.

While most renal embolization procedures can be performed using standard catheterization laboratories, digital subtraction X-ray fluoroscopy, road mapping, biplane angiography and three dimensional (3-D) angiography may be useful in selected patients [2]. Some centers routinely obtain computed tomographic images prior to and/or following embolization procedures.

Embolization Agents

Several types of materials are available for transcatheter renal artery embolization, including metallic coils, sclerosants (liquids), and particulate embolic material. Selecting the type of embolic material depends on the vascular anatomy and hemodynamics, the disease process (pathology) being treated, and the endpoints desired (both technical and clinical) by the operator. The end points may be (a) Embolization (flow reduction/occlusion) of large vessel (b) embolization of end-artery/devascularizing the regional vascular bed), or (c) sclerosis of vascular lesion or vascular bed. Coils or detachable balloons are required for the first end point, particulate or sclerosant (liquid/foam) embolic agents for the second end point, and for the third, a sclerosant is required. The end point can be classified as (1) large vessel/lesion flow reduction/obliteration embolization, (2) end-artery (arteriolar) embolization (devascularizing the regional vascular bed), or (3) sclerosis of vascular lesion or vascular bed.

For the first endpoint, coils and detachable balloons are required; for the second, particulate or sclerosant (liquid/foam) embolic agents are used; and for the third, a sclerosant is required.

Metallic coils may be composed of stainless steel, platinum, or nitinol and some incorporate synthetic fibers for promoting thrombogenicity. Platinum is softer than stainless steel, which allows for tighter packing of coils. Coils are sized according to their core (0.018, 0.035, and 0.038 in.), the diameter of their coil/loop, and the length of the coil. Coils can be deployed using pushable and detachable mechanisms. Pushable coils come preloaded within a sheath, are loaded into the delivery catheter using a wire or a stylette and are delivered using a guidewire or by forceful injection of saline. Detachable coils, such as the popular Gugleimi coil (Boston Scientific, Natick, MA), are released via electrolysis of a stainless steel connector. Other detachable coils include the AZUR coils (Terumo, Japan) and the interlock coils (Boston Scientific, Natick, MA). Detachable balloons are less commonly used for renal artery embolization because of a higher failure rate owing to their propensity to deform and deflate. They are occasionally used in high-flow, large-caliber arteriovenous fistulae or large aneurysms.

Particulate embolization agents can be composed of either biodegradable (gelfoam) or permanent materials, such as polyvinyl alcohol (PVA) and embospheres. Gelfoam is ideal for benign post-traumatic hemorrhage or to minimize blood loss pre-operatively for tumor resection/nephrectomy. It is the least expensive of embolic materials and has a less permanent embolic effect, usually lasting for 2–3 weeks, although a permanent embolic effect can be achieved with gelfoam secondary although an inflammatory response or formation of an organized thrombus may cause permanent occlusion. For general applications of renal artery embolization, satisfactory PVA particles have an irregular surface and a tendency to clump within the delivery catheters, clogging the catheter/microcatheter or resulting in larger sized clumps of particles. In contrast, embospheres (trisacryl gelatin) permeate deeper into lesions than PVA particles of comparable sizes, resulting in more extensive vascular occlusion. In addition, embospheres are hydrophilic, which reduces clumping even within the catheter. Consequently, this agent is becoming more popular for renal artery embolization.

Liquid agents include *N*-butyl-2-cyanoacrylate glue, 98–99 % ethanol, ethibloc, bucrylate, Sotradecol foam.

Since these agents are not radiopaque, they are often mixed with Lipiodol or other contrast media prior to embolization. Liquid agents penetrate deeper than particulate agents and coils, and hence should be used with caution. Ethanol is a sclerosing agent that penetrates to the capillary bed, devitalizing the vascular bed and is useful for large-area tissue destruction. Cardiopulmonary collapse is a rare but dire complication of Ethanol injection, and great care should be taken to limit the quantity of alcohol injected. It should be avoided in patients with pulmonary hypertension. If feasible, it may be desirable to occlude the parent artery for a few minutes during tissue ablation, followed by aspiration of residual alcohol. These agents are not radiopaque and can achieve deeper penetration than particulate and coil embolization, and therefore should be used with caution. Ethanol is a sclerosing agent that passes through the capillary circulation and is useful for large-area tissue destruction.

Partial Versus Total Embolization

When it is desirable to eliminate the vascular supply to a portion of the kidney while minimizing the extent of infarction of the functional portions of the kidney, partial renal artery embolization techniques are used.

This is achieved with selective catheterization of segmental/lobar renal artery branches that perfuse a lesion.

Superselective embolization can provide controlled occlusion of specific small renal artery branches that supply blood to a lesion, with very little effect on the surrounding normal renal parenchyma. One study reported less than 10 % of nontarget renal parenchymal infarction using superselective renal artery embolization, which was not associated with a clinically significant reduction in renal function. In contrast, subselective embolization resulted in >15–50 % infarction of the surrounding renal parenchyma, which may compromise renal function. In any event, the patient should be made aware before the procedure that there is always a risk for nontarget embolization and that some normal renal parenchyma may need to be sacrificed to accomplish the intended goal. This is because the vessels in the kidney are "end arteries" with no significant intrarenal collaterals.

When the goal is total renal infarction or total obliteration of blood supply to tumors which occupy most of the renal parenchyma, total renal artery embolization techniques should be preferred. This is achieved by positioning the catheter within the main renal artery but distal to the ostium to minimize reflux into the aorta and cause spinal, lower extremity, and bowel infarction. Embolization of small arterial branches with alcohol, polyvinyl alcohol (PVA) particles, microspheres, and/or Gelfoam is performed until there is contrast stasis in the targeted kidney. After flushing the guiding catheter, coils may be deployed in the main renal artery. Coils may occasionally be used as the sole embolization agent, provided total cessation of flow can be documented. For performing superselective renal artery embolization a 4F or 5F catheter is first positioned into the main renal artery or its primary branches and angiography done to identify the target vessel. Through this catheter, a 2F/3F microcatheter is inserted over a 0.018 or 0.014 inch guidewire which is positioned in the target branch vessel. It is important to flush the larger lumen catheter at regular intervals to prevent thrombus formation. The embolization material (e.g. PVA particles, Gelfoam particles or Embospheres) is then cautiously injected taking care to prevent reflux into a non-target vessel. Embolisation is continued till sluggish flow or contrast stasis is noted. If ethanol is being used for embolization, a balloon occlusion catheter is often positioned initially in the proximal or parent artery to prevent reflux. If necessary coils may be deployed in the parent vessel via the microcatheter (0.018 inch coils) or the outer catheter (0.035 inch coils). Pushable coils are commonly used owing to their ease of deployment and lower cost compared to detachable coils.

Superselective renal artery embolization.

Combined/Complex Techniques

Patients with wide necked aneurysms may require more advanced or complex procedures like the remodeling and balloon assisted techniques [5, 6]. The remodeling technique consists of deploying a bare stent across the aneurysm neck after superselective catheterization of the aneurysm. Subsequently, embolization material typically coils are introduced into the aneurysm sac, while the stent in the parent artery serves as a scaffold, preventing coil migration. Balloon-assisted embolization involves superselective catheterization of the aneurysm, followed by transient inflation of the balloon in the parent artery across the aneurysm neck, when embolization is performed.

However, this technique usually involves the use of large (8F) sheaths or bilateral vascular access.

Renal Transplants

The most common indications for embolization in patients after renal transplantation are for the treatment of an arteriovenous fistula (AVF) or pseudoaneurysms.

AVFs almost always occur as a result of percutaneous biopsies of the allograft, reported to occur in 1–18 % of cases [7, 8]. To a lesser extent, percutaneous nephrostomy tube placements have also been reported as a cause for AVF formation. RAE is considered the first line of treatment for symptomatic AVF [9]. Pseudoaneurysms can occur in up to 30 % of biopsied allografts and can also be treated with transcatheter coil embolization.

Since the transplanted kidney is most often anastomosed to the external or internal iliac artery, the techniques for embolization of lesions in renal allografts require some modification. Non-selective angiography is often necessary to visualize the location and origin of the transplant renal artery. Carbon dioxide may be used for angiography to reduce the risk of nephrotoxicity and because it has a higher sensitivity for detecting small AVF [10]. Depending on the location and orientation of the transplant kidney artery, an ipsilateral or contralateral femoral artery approach may be used. Coaxial techniques may be necessary in selected cases with tortuous vessels or unusual orientation of the renal artery. After the aortic bifurcation is traversed with the guidewire, the catheter can be exchanged for a hydrophilic catheter and superselective methods with coaxial systems may be implemented to access the lesion better.

Several studies report minor infarcts (<30 % of allograft) occurring in up to 100 % of cases involving coil embolization of lesions, but no data on the long-term consequences with regard to allograft survival have yet been reported in the literature [11]. In one series, in 28.6 % of patients, 30–50 % infarction of the allograft has been reported [12].

Unlike in native kidneys, to maximize the function of the renal allograft, complete obliteration of the AVF or pseudoaneurysm is not necessary unless symptoms persist, in which case repeat microcoil embolization can be done. If the feeding vessel of a pseudoaneurysm cannot be accessed through the transplant renal artery, transcapsular embolization of the pseudoaneurysm can be attempted with optimal operator experience [13].

Embolization for Malignant Tumours

The most common indication for renal artery embolization is preoperative infarction of renal tumors prior to nephrectomy or radiofrequency ablation (RFA) [14, 15].

RAE can be used for palliation by reducing the tumor bulk and providing symptomatic (hematuria, flank pain) relief in patients with unresectable renal cell carcinoma or in patients who are poor surgical candidates (Fig. 4.3).

By decreasing the size and vascularity of the tumor, RAE also allows for a less-extensive surgical resection and decreased intraoperative blood loss [16, 17]. Several studies have also demonstrated that RAE-induced tumor necrosis may stimulate a tumor specific response, and further decrease its size preoperatively. RAE increases the edema within the tissue planes between the tumor and kidney, which makes dissection easier in patients who under go nephrectomy [17, 18]. This added benefit is most pronounced at 72 h following RAE. In cases where there is a large burden of tumor thrombus, the time taken to maximize the decrease in tumor size may be longer than 72 h. This benefit must be weighed against the increased chance of collateral vessel formation which occurs within 72 h. Therefore, it has been recommended that the ideal time between RAE and surgery is less than 24 h to 2 days. One pilot study also has reported preprocedural infarction of renal tumors prior to cryoablation reduces the size of the postcryoablation hematoma [19].

Technical success can be achieved using a variety of embolization agents. After selection or superselection of the artery or arteries feeding the tumor, ethanol mixed with lipiodol, PVA particles, synthetic microspheres, or Gelfoam can be used to occlude the capillaries of the tumor for patients planned for a partial or total nephrectomy. If a total nephrectomy is planned, coil embolization of the main renal artery and any extrarenal feeding vessels should be performed. The use of sclerosants should be done with caution as normal renal parenchyma can be affected and injury to surrounding results can result from inadvertent reflux.

A residual stump of the proximal renal artery should be spared to allow surgical clamping and ligation during the total nephrectomy without the problem of metallic coils hindering resection of the main renal artery or migrating back into the aorta and embolizing distally.

If there is a large amount of shunting within the tumor, coils or Gelfoam can be used to block them. Gelfoam when coupled with sealing coils has been reported to achieve stasis for 24–72 h, which is the usual time lapse between embolization and subsequent nephrectomy. After embolization, a completion aortogram is then performed to evaluate for accessory or parasitized arteries that may be supplying the tumor.

Repeat embolization may be performed as necessary. Superselection of the feeding arteries for a renal tumor is preferred in patients planned for RFA and cryoablation.

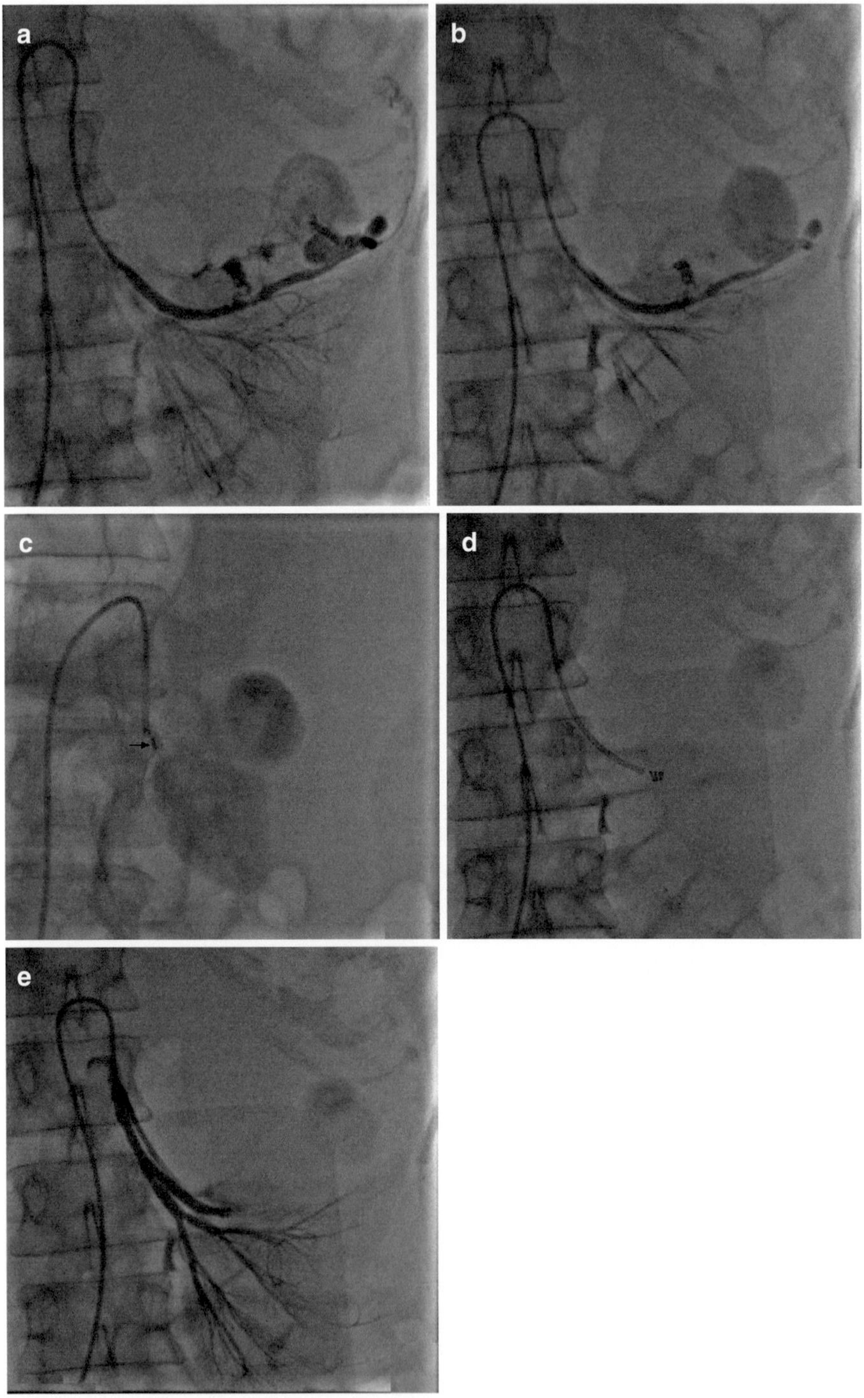

Fig. 4.3 (**a**–**e**) Renal pseudoaneurysm with hematuria following trauma which was embolized using a single coil (*arrow*)

Preoperative RAE may be advantageous in patients with stage 1 renal cell carcinoma planned for RFA, possibly due to the devascularized region having a reduced heat sump effect, thus rendering RFA more effective.

Long-Term benefits Although its long-term effects are controversial, one study reports an increased overall 5-year survival benefit for patients that undergo prenephrectomy RAE compared with patients who undergo nephrectomy alone (62 % vs. 35 %; P=0.01) [20]. To date, there is no prospective data reported to demonstrate a survival benefit to adjuvant RAE prior to nephrectomy [21, 22].

Renal Angiomyolipomas

Renal angiomyolipomas are benign vascular tumors that contain fat and smooth muscle elements. Tumors larger than 4 cm in diameter are at greater than 50 % risk of rupture and hemorrhage. Transcatheter renal artery embolization is now the treatment of choice for acute hemorrhage from angiomyolipomas and may eliminate the need for blood transfusion and surgery in technically successful cases. A decrease in tumor size can also be seen in nonhemorrhagic angiomyolipomas that undergo RAE [23, 24].

Technical success can be achieved with several embolic agents. Embolic agents commonly used are microcoils, nonresorbable particles, absolute dehydrated ethanol (typically mixed with an oily contrast agent such as Ethiodol), Sotradecol, and N-butyl-2-cyanoacrylate [25].

Given that angiomyolipomas are quite vascular, liquid embolic agents/sclerosants such as absolute dehydrated alcohol mixed with an oily contrast agent such as Ethiodol, Sotradecol, and glue have been recommended over particulate embolic agents and coils in some centres. There is virtually no loss of renal function in the reported cases of treated AMLs with RAE. Although technical success has been reported to be in 80–90 % of cases using superselective methods, long-term follow-up has shown tumor recurrence in over 30 % of patients, with a higher recurrence rate of 43 % in tuberous sclerosis patients [26, 27]. For this reason, these patients should undergo continued surveillance and proper counseling for potential future recurrences after RAE. One study reports angiomyolipomas undergo sterile liquefaction after RAE, sometimes requiring percutaneous drainage catheter placement [27].

Traumatic Renal Hemorrhage

Renal injuries in the setting of abdominal trauma are not uncommon. The most frequent presenting sign is hematuria or perinephric hematoma, but the amount of bleeding is usually a poor indicator of the severity of the trauma. The majority of renal artery injuries are minor (75–80 %), representing contusions or superficial lacerations that can be managed conservatively, with only 5 % grade V (completely shattered kidney or an avulsed renal hilum that devascularizes the kidney). The remaining 10 % are generally serious injuries that are amenable to renal artery embolization [28]. Early diagnosis and treatment is necessary to preserve the maximum amount of normal renal tissue, as renal ischemia persisting for 3 h or more may result in severe tubular necrosis and renal dysfunction. Additionally, a delay in diagnosis may result in an increased deformity of the kidney due to a large hematoma, which can prevent superselective catheter placement, therefore necessitating a more proximal embolization resulting in more parenchymal loss due to infarction.

Wide impact injuries that result in a broad volume of parenchymal injury should be evaluated first with CT for grading purposes, if the patient is stable. These injuries include stab and gunshot wounds, blunt trauma, and deceleration injuries, which can avulse the main renal arteries due to the relatively mobile kidneys that stretch the renal vessels. Higher-grade renal injuries or unstable patients may need to be operated on emergently.

Interventional procedures may be indicated in more stable patients as well as in postoperative patients with persistent or recurrent hematuria [28, 29].

Narrow tract injuries from assaults, biopsies, and nephrostomy tube placements leave more sharply defined residual wound tracts. Not only can arterial injury occur in these settings, but also false aneurysms with or without arteriovenous fistulas. The exact location of vessel damage can be assessed with CT, but direct angiography is more likely to be definitive in these cases. Although most cases of arterial injuries after biopsy or nephrostomy tube placement heal spontaneously, if hematuria persists for longer than 3 days, angiographic investigation and possible embolization is warranted. Patients who become hemodynamically unstable following biopsies and nephrostomy should undergo immediate angiography and treatment [30].

Most injuries resulting from biopsy or nephrostomy tube placements have been treated primarily with embolization, therefore avoiding surgery.

Agents used include Gelfoam because of its utility and absorbability in small vessel injuries, PVA particles, or microcoils for larger vessel injuries. A success rate of 93 % has been reported in the literature for emergent hemorrhage cases. Precise selection and embolization of peripheral lesions with the use of coaxial catheters is preferred to preserve as much kidney function as possible.

Arteriovenous Fistulas

Arteriovenous fistulas are rare lesions, often seen as a result of biopsies of native and transplanted kidneys, partial nephrectomy, percutaneous nephrostomy tube placement, and penetrating trauma [30]. Although 70 % of AVFs in renal allografts spontaneously resolve within 2 years, embolization is the treatment of choice for symptomatic AVFs [31, 32]. Patients usually present with hematuria, abdominal bruit, renal insufficiency, hypertension, and high output cardiac failure. Endovascular management is preferred over surgery to preserve renal function [2, 7]. Even large, high-flow renal AVFs have been successfully treated with RAE.

Technical success can be achieved with superselective catheters with coaxial systems to embolize the fistulous tract with microcoils. Particles are not utilized in AVF as they pose a risk of passing through the connection between the artery and vein, which could lead to embolization in the pulmonary circulation [33, 34]. On diagnostic angiography, there is early opacification of the vein, nearly simultaneous with the adjacent artery confirming the presence of an AVF. If the fistula is chronic, the artery and vein may be dilated due to increased flow. There may be extravasation of contrast into the renal collecting system in the presence of an arteriocalyceal fistula. Complete obliteration of the fistula tract is the technical goal. In cases of renal allografts, control of patient symptoms should be the desired goal instead in order to preserve as much functional renal parenchyma as possible. To achieve this, crossing through the fistula from the arterial side to the venous side is ideal to deposit the coil through the fistula. In cases where there is high arterial blood flow, a balloon can be used to temporarily occlude the draining vein and prevent coils from entering the systemic circulation.

Renal Artery Pseudoaneurysm

Renal artery pseudoaneurysms are also uncommon, seen in patients after a renal biopsy, partial nephrectomy, or trauma. Most of the time, they are asymptomatic when small and spontaneously thrombose [35]. However, when they are symptomatic, a patient can present with a pulsatile mass in the pelvis, flank pain and renal dysfunction secondary to compression of artery branches or shunting of blood, or hemorrhage from rupture. Although these lesions can be managed surgically, RAE is preferred if they are amenable to embolization to minimize the loss of normal functioning renal parenchyma.

Technical success can be achieved with superselective catheters to embolize the pseudoaneurysm with microcoils or stents. On angiography, they appear as localized segments of arterial dilatation. If acute, they have a smooth contour and when chronic, they have an irregular contour. To minimize the risk of compromising the distal renal artery flow, a narrow pseudoaneurysm neck is ideal for embolization procedures [36, 37].

In cases where the main renal artery is affected, to avoid devascularizing of the entire kidney, one could consider the use of covered stents to exclude the pseudoaneurysm. The success rates for transcatheter treatment of pseudoaneurysms range from 71 to 100 % with alleviation of symptoms in 57–88 % of cases [33, 34].

Arteriovenous Malformation

Arteriovenous malformations (AVMs) of the kidney, which are rare, are typically described as moderate to high flow, and can be congenital or acquired. Congenital AVMs are usually small and asymptomatic, and close spontaneously. Acquired

AVMs typically have an indolent, complex course. When they are symptomatic, patients usually present with gross hematuria, renal dysfunction, hypertension, and high-output cardiac failure [38, 39].

Because of their complexity, these lesions are almost never entirely cured and may recur. Patients with these lesions should be counseled that treatment may be lifelong and that currently there is no permanant cure. Therefore, the endpoint is not to completely obliterate the vascular anomaly seen on angiography, but to reverse the clinical symptoms and repeat embolizations as needed [11, 12].

The optimal method of improving patient symptoms is to ablate the nidus of the AVM, which is the epicenter of the abnormal vessels. For this reason, sclerosants are preferred over coils and detachable balloons that are not fine enough to negotiate the nidus. Because of the moderate to high flow in these AVMs, more-viscous sclerosants such as N-butyl-2-cyanoacrylate (glue), Onyx, and Sotradecol/CO_2 foam can be used as opposed to alcohol, which can be more difficult to control in this setting. Gelfoam is not desirable in the treatment for AVMs because of its temporary embolic effect and risk of recanalization of the nidus. A balloon-occlusion catheter can be placed proximal to the lesion to decrease the flow into the nidus, so that the sclerosant can dwell and not pass through a high-flow fistula. Epinephrine injection before embolization may also make the procedure more effective by inducing vasoconstriction, thereby concentrating the injected material within the AVM [5, 40, 41].

Coils can also be used in the emergent setting to rapidly reduce blood flow in patients who are actively bleeding, as well as to reduce symptoms and the risk of preoperative bleeding before partial or total nephrectomy.

Renal Artery Aneurysm

Renal artery aneurysms are rare lesions, with a prevalence of 0.7 % based on CT imaging of the general population [34]. Predisposing factors include atherosclerosis and connective tissue diseases such as Marfan syndrome and Ehlers-Danlos syndrome, neurofibromatosis, fibromuscular dysplasia, polyarteritis nodosa, and tuberous sclerosis.

Although there are no definite indications for aneurysm treatment, in general, aneurysms greater than 1.5–2.0 cm in diameter, or aneurysms presenting with flank pain, hematuria, found in women of child-bearing age or in patients with polyarteritis nodosa warrant intervention.

Embolization has resulted in 100 % technical success and resolution of symptoms in 88 % of patients with extraparenchymal renal artery aneurysms [42]. The location and morphology of the aneurysms determines the particular technique needed for embolization. Main renal artery aneurysms are more amenable to stent grafting alone. However, the proximal-most aspect of the stent must be at least 1.5 mm away from the renal artery ostium and first bifurcation. Vessel tortuosity and angulations may limit the use of a stent graft despite the advent of more flexible devices. Distal renal artery branch aneurysms are more likely to be amenable to coil embolization with superselective catheterization.

Aneurysms with a wide neck, which can be defined as greater than 70 % of the diameter of the aneurysm may require advanced techniques using a combination of a stent graft or balloon occlusion device with coils [42, 43].

Chronic Renal Parenchymal Diseases

Chronic renal parenchymal disease such as end-stage renal disease, posttransplant patients with severe nephrotic syndrome, hypertension or hematuria, persistent urine leak from a ureterocutaneous fistula, severe and intractable hydronephrosis, autosomal dominant polycystic kidney disease, and irreversible transplant rejection have been reported indications for complete renal artery embolization in patients who may be poor surgical candidates for nephrectomy [1, 44, 45]. The goal is to provide symptomatic relief by eliminating renal function while avoiding the morbidity and mortality of a nephrectomy.

Technical success can best be achieved using liquid or particulate agents to initially embolize small peripheral arteries, and coils to embolize large vessels. It is therefore crucial to know the number of renal arteries that supply the kidney as well as the presence of aberrant arteries. In chronically diseased transplant kidneys or in end-stage renal disease, the renal arteries may be small, which predisposes to reflux of embolization material into the aorta. It is for this reason that temporary balloon occlusion catheters can be positioned in the proximal main renal artery to avoid this problem. Certain technical improvisations may be required such as avoiding brisk injections of embolizing agents and cessation of injection when vascular stasis occurs. The endpoint is to observe stasis of contrast or slow to-and-fro flow in the main renal artery on completion angiography. Repeat embolization can be performed as needed.

Complications of RAE

Renal artery embolization is considered a safe procedure, with a relatively low complication rate. The most common occurrence is the postembolization syndrome that affects over 90 % of patients. Patients usually present with mild flank pain, fever, nausea, vomiting, paralytic ileus, and/or leucocytosis for 1–3 days after RAE [46]. Treatment is supportive, consisting of analgesics, antipyretics, and antiemetics as needed, until symptoms resolve, typically within few days. For this reason, it is recommended that patients be observed in a hospital overnight after RAE for monitoring and symptom control.

Coil migration is an unusual, but potentially serious, complication, occurring in less than 2 % of cases. Typically, this is detected at the end of the embolization procedure and can be rectified using an endovascular grasping device (snare). Inadvertent nontarget embolization can result in spine, lower extremity, and bowel infarction. Reflux of embolization materials can result in loss of renal function and subsequent hypertension and inadvertent passage of PVA particles through an AVF can result in pulmonary embolism [47, 48].

Positioning the injection catheter properly and securely, possibly with the use of a temporary balloon occlusion device within the parent artery can reduce this risk. Finally, contrast nephrotoxicity can occur, especially in those with limited renal function, and this should be considered when planning the procedure [15, 49].

The incidence of infection related to RAE is very low. Follow-up imaging may demonstrate the presence of intrarenal gas, but this does not necessarily indicate infection. There have been only a few reported cases of post-RAE patients requiring a percutaneous drainage catheter [49].

Nephrostomy Tubes

The presence of nephrostomy tubes does not interfere with the renal artery embolization. However, it is recommended to flush the nephrostomy with saline and instill gentamicin after the procedure [48].

Familiarity with the appearance of expected RAE changes of the kidney on cross-sectional imaging on CT is important to avoid unnecessary interventions [49].

Our Experience in Renal Artery Embolization

In our Institution, we have performed renal artery embolization in a variety of clinical situations from 2003 to 2016. There were 23 patients who had undergone the procedure for a variety of indications listed below.

Embolization for Pseudo Aneurysms, Urological Injuries, Post Renal Biopsy Injury and Stab Injury

There were five patients with iatrogenic renal injuries who presented with hematuria, listed in Table 4.1. The mean age of the patients was 32 ± 9.8 years. There were three females. Their mean hemoglobin was 5.2 ± 3.2 g/ dl. All patients presented with hematuria requiring blood transfusions. There were two patients who were hemodynamically unstable following multiple stab injuries. Angiography revealed arterivenous fistulas in all patients. The patients presenting with multiple stab injuries had multiple arteriovenous fistulas (Fig. 4.5a–c). Two patients had arteriovenous fistulas following renal biopsies, while one patient developed arteriovenous

Table 4.1 Characterization of patients, lesion type, cause and catheters used along with embolizing agents used for renal artery embolizations

Age/Sex	Lesion type/number/ site	Cause	Catheter/embolizingagent
Renal artery embolization for Renal Injuries:			
40/M	AVF	2 percutaneous nephrostomy, insertion for hydronephrosis	Judkins Right/PVA
56/F	AVF 1	Biopsy	Judkins Right/ PVA
45/M	AVF 4	Stab injury	Judkins Right/PVA
9/F	AVF 1	Biopsy	Judkins Right/Coils
40/F	AVF 6/ pseudoaneurysm	Stab injury	Judkins Right/ Coils
Renal artery embolization for angiolipomas/ renal cell carcinomas:			
52/F	Extravasation	Angiolipoma	5 F Cobra/ PVA
30/M	Pseudoaneurysm	Angiolipoma	4 F Vertebral/ coils
46/F	Perinephric hematoma	Angiolipoma	5 F Cobra/ PVA
80 M	Extravasations	Renal cell carcinoma	5 F Cobra/ coils
76/M	Extravasations	Renal cell carcinoma	5 F Cobra/ Gel Foam
67/F	Extravasations	Renal cell carcinoma	Judkins Right/ coils
75/M	Extravasations	Renal cell carcinoma	5 F Cobra/ coils
45/M	Pseudoaneurysm	Angiolipoma	5 F Cobra/ PVA
55/M	Extravasations	APKD, ESRD	6 F Reuter/ Gel Foam
Renal artery embolization for resistant hypertension in ESRD:			
47/M	Renal artery	Resistant HTN/ESRD	6 F Judkins Right/ coils
56/F	Renal artery	Resistant HTN/ESRD	6 F Judkins Right/ coils
45/M	Renal artery	Resistant HTN/ESRD	6 F Judkins Right/ coils
65/F	Renal artery	Resistant HTN/ESRD	6 F Judkins/GelFoam
55/M	Renal artery	Resistant HTN/ESRD	6 F Judkins/Gel Foam
12/F	Hypoplastic distal renal arteries	Resistant HTN S/p Renal Transplant	5 F Judkins/ coils
20/F	Rt. Renal artery stenosis	Resistant HTN/ abortions	5 F Judkins/ coils
			After renal angioplasty
Renal artery embolization for resistant proteinuria and edema in ESRD:			
9/M	Renal artery	Resistant proteinuria/ ESRD	5 F IMA/PVA
45/M	Renal artery	Resistant proteinuria/ ESRD	6 F Judkins/Gel Foam

AVF arteriovenous fistula, *HTN* hypertension, *APKD* adult polycystic kidney disease, *ESRD* end stage renal disease, *PVA* poly vinyl alcohol, *IMA* internal mammary artery catheter

fistulas following a percutaneous nephrostomy insertion for hydronephrosis (Figs. 4.3, 4.4, 4.5, 4.6, and 4.7).

Selective angiography of the culprit renal artery was usually done using a 5 F/ 6F Judkins Right coronary catheter (Cordis Corporation, Tipperary, Ireland) through a

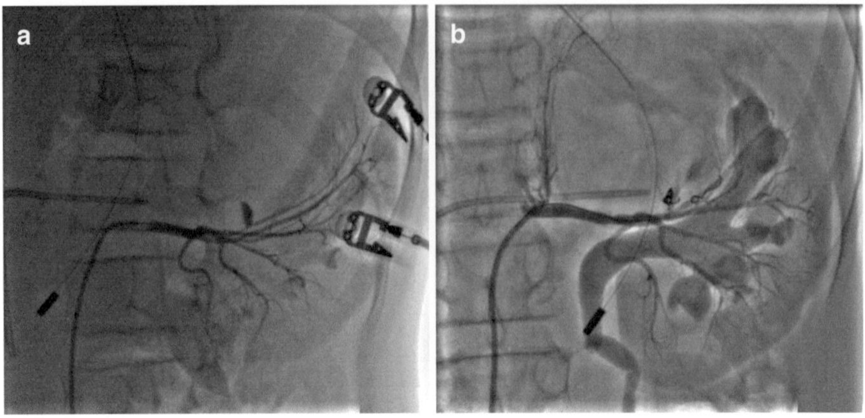

Fig. 4.4 (**a**, **b**) Pseudoaneurysm of a branch renal artery secondary to pancreatitis and pseudocyst (note the mass effect on the upper pole of the kidney). This was embolised using a microcatheter and micro coils

6 F right femoral artery sheath. The culprit renal artery was identified by the presence of abnormal arteriovenous communications or extravasation of dye. The catheter or microcatheter was advanced as near aspossible to the lesion, and the embolizing agent was injected. Whenever the culprit vessel could be superselectively cannulated using a co-axially placed micro catheter (Tracker, Boston Scientific, Natick, Massachusetts, USA), micro coils (2 × 20 mm) or Cook's embolization coils (35-2-3 to 35-5-5) (M Reye ® Embolization coil, Cook Incorporated, Bloomington, IN, USA) were used to embolize the lesion.

Whenever the culprit vessel and the size of the fistula was small, 700 μ Poly Vinyl Alcohol (PVA) particles (Cook Incorporated, Bloomington, IN, USA) or Gel Foam shavings (Ab Gel, Sri Gopal Krishna Labs Pvt. Ltd. Kandivali (W), Mumbai, India) mixed with contrast agent and saline was injected. Injection of embolizing material was stopped when the distal vessels were embolized and flow became sluggish. Care was taken to prevent reflux of dye with particles, by avoiding aggressive injection [4]. The catheter should be gently flushed with saline before performing check angiography.

Complete cessation of renovascular bleeding after the embolization procedure was defined as technical success. Resolution of gross hematuria, absence of recurrent hematuria, no recurrent need for blood transfusion, no recurrent decrease of hemoglobin, and absence of need for angiographic re-embolization or subsequent renal surgery were regarded as medical success. Non-target embolization of vascular territories, iatrogenic vascular damage, and puncture-site bleeding were labelled as technical complications. Medical complications included post-embolization syndrome (back pain and fever not otherwise accounted for), perirenal abscess or renal abscess, decrease in renal function, and arterial hypertension.

Technical success was achieved in all patients and medical success was achieved in two. There were no complications of non-target vessel embolization. One patient developed post-embolization syndrome. None developed peri renal or renal abscess, decrease in renal function or hypertension.

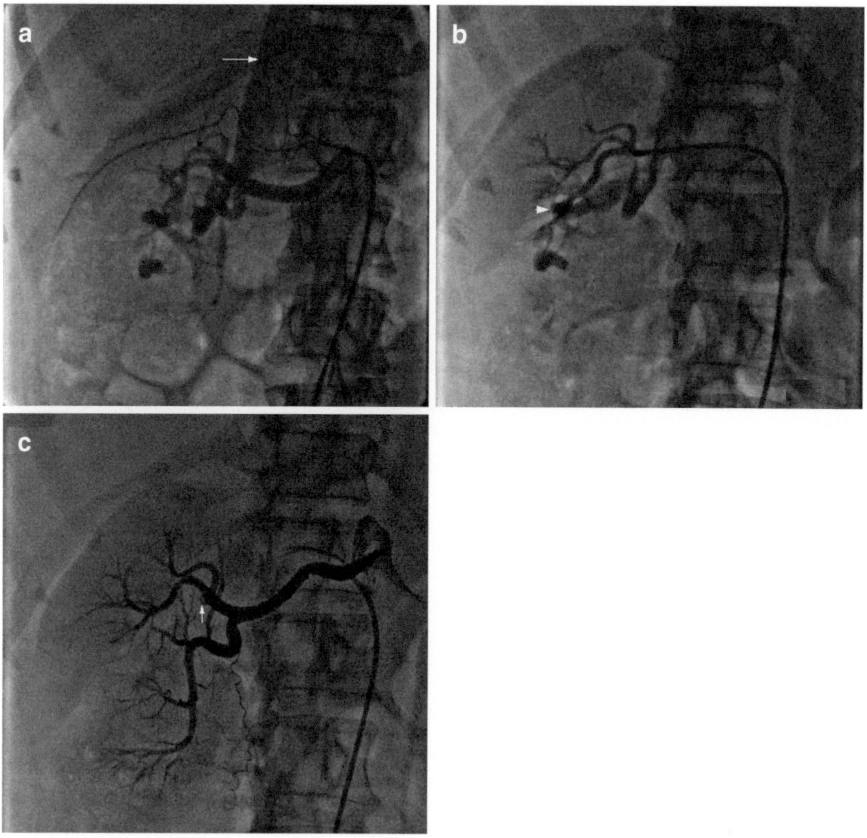

Fig. 4.5 Renal angiograms of a patient with traumatic AVM due to stab injury showing (**a**) early opacifiation of Inferior Vena Cava (*arrow*). Selective angiogram (**b**) showing location of AVM (*arrow-head*) and (**c**) coil occlusion (*arrow*) of the feeding artery of the AVM

Persistent Hematuria Due to Inoperable Renal Cell Carcinoma, Angiolipoma and Polycystic Kidneys

Indications for embolization are preoperative devascularisation to ease resection and decrease blood loss, palliative therapy in patients with unresectable tumor or who are not surgical candidates, and treatment of hemorrhagic complications. There were four patients with angiolipoma and four patients with renal cell carcinoma requiring devascularisation (Table 4.1).

The mean age of patients with angiolipoma was 45 ± 5 years, with two females. Their mean hemoglobin was 12 ± 4.5 g/dl with normal creatinine values; mean creatinine of 0.8 ± 0.02 mg/dl. Renal angiography revealed extravasations in two patients while one had a pseudoaneurysm and one presented with a perinephric hematoma. The patient with the pseudoaneurysm required selective cannulation of the feeder vessel with a 4 F vertebral catheter and subsequent embolization with Cook's coils 35-4-4.

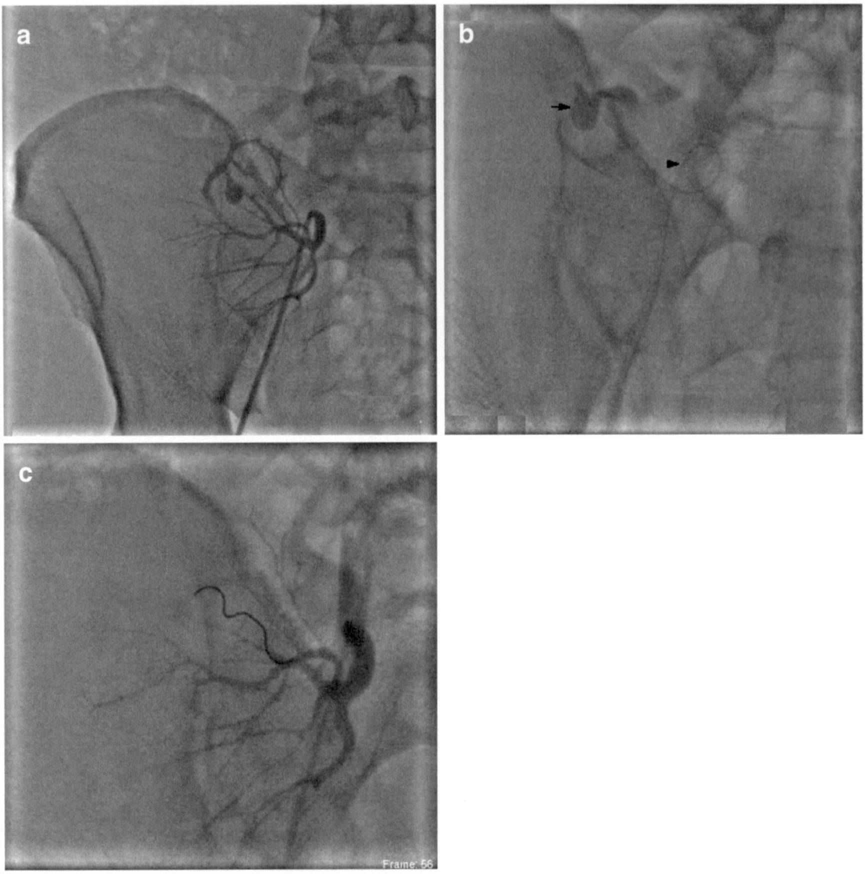

Fig. 4.6 (**a**, **b**) Arteriovenous fistula within the parenchyma of a transplanted kidney following renal biopsy. Microcatheter (*arrowhead*) advanced to the site of AVM (*arrow*) and (**c**) embolisation of the feeding branch using PVA particles and coils

When the angiolipoma was large measuring >10 cms, the renal artery was selectively cannulated and advanced as near the tumour blush using 5 F Simons or 5 F Cobra catheters (Terumo Glidecath, Terumo Medical Corporation, Somerset, NJ, USA) and PVA particles of 350–700 μ were injected with successful embolization of the renal artery branch (Fig. 4.4).

As the renal cell carcinoma in all four patients affected almost the whole kidney, the ipsilateral renal artery was cannulated using a 5 F Cobra catheter and 3 × 4 cms and 4 × 4 cms Cook coils were deployed into it embolizing the renal artery. In some patients, Gel Foam was used to embolize the renal artery. The choice of embolization material was based on the caliber of the renal arteries supplying the tumor as well as financial considerations (Gel foam is very inexpensive). Total occlusion was

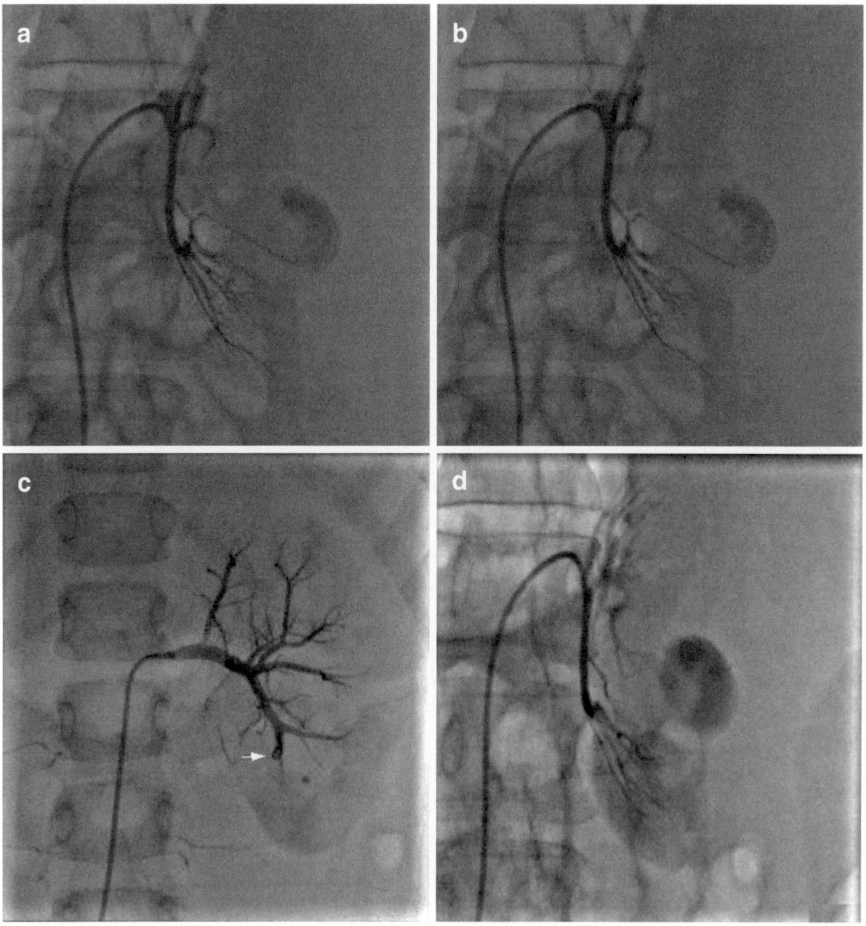

Fig. 4.7 Embolization of an AVM following renal biopsy. Selective angiography shows a narrow high pressure jet into a large pseudoaneurysm (**a**). Following selective cannulation, the feeding artery was embolised using a coil (**b**) with successful obliteration of the pseudoaneurysm (**c**). Note that the renal parenchymais distorted due to perinephric hematoma

confirmed by angiography following embolization. All these patients had normal creatinine values; with a mean creatinine of 0.9 ± 0.03 mg/dl. All patients presented with hematuria with a mean hemoglobin of 9.8 ± 1.6 g/dl.

Technical success was achieved in all patients. The patient with inoperable renal cell carcinoma with persistent hematuria had total cessation of hematuria at 48 h following the procedure. The patients with angiolipoma demonstrated significant decrease in tumor vascularity and underwent successful nephrectomy few weeks to a month later. None of these patients demonstrated non-target vessel embolization. None had procedure related medical complications.

Renal Embolization for Refractory Hypertension Due to Renal Artery Stenosis

There were seven patients with end stage renal disease (ESRD) Stage V on maintenance hemodialysis and planned for renal transplantation, presenting with resistant hypertension uncontrolled with 5 ± 3.5 anti-hypertensive medications (Table 4.1).

Their mean age was 39 ± 12 years, with four females. The mean blood pressure before the procedure was 180 ± 18 mmHg systolic and 99 ± 6 mmHg diastolic. The mean creatinine was 8.9 ± 3.5 mg/dl. They all had contracted kidneys and some had renal artery stenosis. They were cannulated using 6 F/ 5 F Right Judkins catheters and were embolized using Gel Foam or 35-3-4 Cook's coils. Repeat angiography confirmed total occlusion of bilateral renal arteries.

In one female patient with resistant hypertension and recurrent abortions due to pre-eclampsia, renal angiography revealed a normal left kidney with a severely stenosed right renal artery supplying a contracted right kidney. Since stable catheter position could not be achieved, angioplasty of the right renal artery was initially performed using 2 × 10 mm and 2.5 × 10 mm balloons to enlarge the stenotic lumen. Following this a 5F Right Judkins catheter could be advanced deep within the artery and 3 Cook coils measuring 35-2-3, 35-3-3 and 35-5-5 were deployed. An early arising upper pole renal artery could not be coil embolized due to its small caliber and was embolized using 180–300 μ PVA particles. Total occlusion of right renal artery was confirmed by repeat angiography.

Following renal transplantation, a 12 year old female presented with resistant hypertension. Selective angiography of the graft kidney revealed normal anastomosis of aorta and normal renal arteries. Selective angiography of the renal arteries done using 5 F right Judkinscatheter revealed normal renal arteries with hypoplastic distal vessels. Therefore, 35-3-4 Cook's coils were deployed in each renal artery resulting in successful occlusion of both renal arteries.

One patient who presented with renal artery stenosis and contracted ipsilateral kidney had technical success with decrease in anti-hypertensive medications following the procedure from three drugs to a single drug. In five patients, technical success was achieved with decrease in the need for anti-hypertensive drugs from 5 ± 3.5 pre-procedure to 1 ± 1 post-procedure. Post-embolization, the blood pressure decreased to 140 ± 4.5 mmHg systolic and 85 ± 4.3 mmHg diastolic. In two patients where only unilateral renal artery embolization was successful, although technical success was achieved, due to incompleteness of the procedure there was no decrease in the anti-hypertensive medications. Post-embolization syndrome developed in one patient. None developed peri renal or renal abscess. Post-infarction syndrome was not seen in these patients as it is milder in ESRD patients as opposed to renal tumours due to renal atrophy and decreased amounts of viable renal tissue.

Renal Embolization for Massive Proteinuria in ESRD

There were two patients presenting with refractory edema due to massive refractory proteinuria and ESRD (Table 4.1).

Although some residual renal function was present in both these patients, they were undergoing regular ultrafiltration for the control of anasarca. Both were prospective candidates for renal transplantation. Bilateral renal artery embolization was done to abolish the massive protein loss due to proteinuria.

In the child, both renal arteries were selectively cannulated using a 5 F IMA catheter and were embolized using 45–100 μ, 300 μ and 700 μ PVA particles. Repeat angiography confirmed bilateral total renal artery embolization.

In the adult male, both renal arteries were selectively cannulated using 6 F right Judkins catheter and embolized successfully using Gel Foam.

Their mean creatinine was 4.5 ± 2.3 mg/dl. Serum albumin was 1 ± 0.6 mg/dl and 24 h urine albumin was 8.8 ± 2 g/ 24 h.

Technical success was achieved and there were no medical complications although both patients had severe loin pain requiring opiate analgesia. Following the procedure, there was cessation of proteinuria with rapid decrease in 24 h urinary protein excretion (From 3 g/24 h to 36 mg/ 24 h) and increase in serum albumin from 1.4–3 mg/dl. Six months following the procedure both patients underwent successful renal transplantation.

Mortality Renal artery embolization was unsuccessful in a patient with adult polycystic kidney disease and ESRD, who was hemodynamically unstable, requiring multiple blood transfusions. Medical success could not be achieved as this patient had significant co-morbidities with sepsis and multi-organ failure requiring ventilation. Two months after the procedure, he continued to deteriorate and died of sepsis and multi organ failure.

None developed any major procedure related complications, in our series.

Conclusion

Renal artery embolization has become an effective, therapeutic and adjuvant tool for many acute and chronic urologic and nephrologic diseases. It can be applied successfully in improving preoperative management of renal tumors prior to nephrectomy, achieving hemostasis in cases of hemorrhage from trauma or from tumors, in treating complications of renal transplantation and biopsies such as arteriovenous fistulas and pseudoaneurysms, and for improving symptoms in patients with chronic renal parenchymal diseases. Depending on the indication and the character of the lesion, different embolic materials and catheters are used for optimal outcomes. Preprocedural planning and careful recognition of complications is essential for procedural success. With improvements in technology and techniques, the indications for RAE may expand, making it vital for the interventionalist to be properly aquainted with the presently available techniques.

References

1. Abath C, Andrade G, Cavalcanti D, et al. Complex renal artery aneurysms: liquids or coils? Tech Vasc Interv Radiol. 2007;10:299–307.
2. Manninen HI, Berg M, Vanninen RL. Stent-assisted coil embolization of wide-necked renal artery bifurcation aneurysms. J Vasc Interv Radiol. 2008;19:487–92.
3. Wallace S, Chuang VP, Swanson D, et al. Embolization of renal carcinoma. Radiology. 1981;138:563–70.
4. Derdeyn C, Graves V, Salamat M, et al. Collagen-coated acrylic microspheres for embolotherapy: in vivo and in vitro characteristics. AJNR Am J Neuroradiol. 1997;18:647–53.
5. Sofocleous CT, Hinrichs C, Hubbi B, et al. Angiographic findings and embolotherapy in renal arterial trauma. Cardiovasc Intervent Radiol. 2005;28:39–47.
6. Clark TW, Sankin A, Becske T, et al. Stent-assisted Gugliemi detachable coil repair of wide-necked renal artery aneurysm using 3-D angiography. Vasc Endovascular Surg. 2007;41:528–32.
7. Diaz-Buxo JA, Kopen DF, Donadio Jr JV. Renal allograft arteriovenous fistula following percutaneous biopsy. J Urol. 1974;112(5):577–80.
8. Merkus JW, Zeebregts CJ, Hoitsma AJ, et al. High incidence of arteriovenous fistula after biopsy of kidney allografts. Br J Surg. 1993;80(3):310–2.
9. Loffroy R, Guiu B, Lambert A, et al. Management of postbiopsy renal allograft arteriovenous fistulas with selective arterial embolization: immediate and long-term outcomes. Clin Radiol. 2008;63(6):657–65.
10. Hedegard W, Saad WE, Davies MG. Management of vascular and nonvascular complications after renal transplantation. Tech Vasc Interv Radiol. 2009;12(4):240–62.
11. Maleux G, Messiaen T, Stockx L, Vanrenterghem Y, Wilms G. Transcatheter embolization of biopsy-related vascular injuries in renal allografts. Long-term technical, clinical and biochemical results. Acta Radiol. 2003;44(1):13–7.
12. Dorffner R, Thurnher S, Prokesch R, et al. Embolization of iatrogenic vascular injuries of renal transplants: immediate and follow-up results. Cardiovasc Intervent Radiol. 1998;21(2):129–34.
13. Sennett CA, Messersmith RN, Yousefzadeh DK, Thistlethwaite Jr JR. Percapsular and percutaneous embolization of renal transplant pseudoaneurysm and AV fistula: case report. Cardiovasc Intervent Radiol. 1989;12(5):270–3.
14. Ginat DT, Saad WE, Turba UC. Transcatheter renal artery embolization: clinical applications and techniques. Tech Vasc Interv Radiol. 2009;12(4):224–39.
15. Schwartz MJ, Smith EB, Trost DW, Vaughan Jr ED. Renal artery embolization: clinical indications and experience from over 100 cases. BJU Int. 2007;99(4):881–6.
16. Kalman D, Varenhorst E. The role of arterial embolization in renal cell carcinoma. Scand J Urol Nephrol. 1999;33(3):162–70.
17. Bakal CW, Cynamon J, Lakritz PS, Sprayregen S. Value of preoperative renal artery embolization in reducing blood transfusion requirements during nephrectomy for renal cell carcinoma. J Vasc Interv Radiol. 1993;4(6):727–31.
18. Klimberg I, Hunter P, Hawkins IF, Drylie DM, Wajsman Z. Preoperative angioinfarction of localized renal cell carcinoma using absolute ethanol. J Urol. 1985;133(1):21–4.

19. Woodrum DA, Atwell TD, Farrell MA, Andrews JC, Charboneau JW, Callstrom MR. Role of intraarterial embolization before cryoablation of large renal tumors: a pilot study. J Vasc Interv Radiol. 2010;21(6):930–6.
20. Ginat DT, Saad WE, Turba UC. Transcatheter renal artery embolization for management of renal and adrenal tumors. Tech Vasc Interv Radiol. 2010;13(2):75–88.
21. Yamakado K, Nakatsuka A, Kobayashi S, et al. Radiofrequency ablation combined with renal arterial embolization for the treatment of unresectable renal cell carcinoma larger than 3.5 cm: initial experience. Cardiovasc Intervent Radiol. 2006;29(3):389–94.
22. Arima K, Yamakado K, Kinbara H, Nakatsuka A, Takeda K, Sugimura Y. Percutaneous radiofrequency ablation with transarterial embolization is useful for treatment of stage 1 renal cell carcinoma with surgical risk: results at 2-year mean follow up. Int J Urol. 2007;14(7):585–90.
23. Mondshine RT, Owens S, Mondschein JI, Cizman B, Stavropoulos SW, Clark TW. Combination embolization and radiofrequency ablation therapy for renal cell carcinoma in the setting of coexisting arterial disease. J Vasc Interv Radiol. 2008;19(4):616–20.
24. Zielinski H, Szmigielski S, Petrovich Z. Comparison of preoperative embolization followed by radical nephrectomy with radical nephrectomy alone for renal cell carcinoma. Am J Clin Oncol. 2000;23(1):6–12.
25. Swanson DA, Johnson DE, von Eschenbach AC, Chuang VP, Wallace S. Angioinfarction plus nephrectomy for metastatic renal cell carcinoma—an update. J Urol. 1983;130(3):449–52.
26. Rimon U, Duvdevani M, Garniek A, et al. Large renal angiomyolipomas: digital subtraction angiographic grading and presentation with bleeding. Clin Radiol. 2006;61(6):520–6.
27. Hamlin JA, Smith DC, Taylor FC, et al. Renal angiomyolipomas: long-term follow-up of embolization for acute hemorrhage. Can Assoc Radiol J. 1997;48(3):191–8.
28. Takebayashi S, Horikawa A, Arai M, Iso S, Noguchi K. Transarterial ethanol ablation for sporadic and non-hemorrhaging angiomyolipoma in the kidney. Eur J Radiol. 2009;72(1):139–45.
29. Dabbeche C, Chaker M, Chemali R, et al. Role of embolization in renal angiomyolipomas. J Radiol. 2006;87(12 Pt 1):1859–67.
30. Ramon J, Rimon U, Garniek A, et al. Renal angiomyolipoma: long-term results following selective arterial embolization. Eur Urol. 2009;55(5):1155–61.
31. Kothary N, Soulen MC, Clark TW, et al. Renal angiomyolipoma: long-term results after arterial embolization. J Vasc Interv Radiol. 2005;16(1):45–50.
32. Soulen MC, Faykus Jr MH, Shlansky-Goldberg RD, Wein AJ, Cope C. Elective embolization for prevention of hemorrhage from renal angiomyolipomas. J Vasc Interv Radiol. 1994;5(4):587–91.
33. Fisher RG, Ben-menachem Y. Angiography and embolization in renal trauma. In: Baum S, editor. Abram's angiography: vascular and interventional radiology. 4th ed. Boston: Little, Brown and Company; 1997. p. 1230–43.
34. Teigen CL, Venbrux AC, Quinlan DM, Jeffs RD. Late massive hematuria as a complication of conservative management of blunt renal trauma in children. J Urol. 1992;147(5):1333–6.
35. Fisher RG, Ben-Menachem Y, Whigham C. Stab wounds of the renal artery branches: angiographic diagnosis and treatment by embolization. AJR Am J Roentgenol. 1989;152(6):1231–5.
36. Cope C, Zeit RM. Pseudoaneurysms after nephrostomy. AJR Am J Roentgenol. 1982;139(2):255–61.
37. Low RN, Jeffrey Jr RB. Intraperitoneal hemorrhage after renal biopsy: a grave prognostic sign. AJR Am J Roentgenol. 1988;151(1):113–4.
38. Ashenburg RJ, Blair RJ, Rivera FJ, Weigele JB. Renal arterial rupture complicating transluminal angioplasty: successful conservative management. Radiology. 1990;174(3 Pt 2):983–5.
39. Somani BK, Nabi G, Thorpe P, McClinton S. Endovascular control of haemorrhagic urological emergencies: an observational study. BMC Urol. 2006;6:27.

40. Nakatani T, Uchida J, Han YS, et al. Renal allograft arteriovenous fistula and large pseudoaneurysm. Clin Transplant. 2003;17(1):9–12.
41. Bach AM, Merton DA, Burke Jr JF, Halpern EJ. Sonographic diagnosis of arteriovenous fistula and pseudoaneurysm after biopsy of a transplanted kidney. J Ultrasound Med. 1993;12(9):545–7.
42. Horwitz MD, Hanbury DC, King CM. Renal artery pseudoaneurysm following partial nephrectomy treated with stent-graft. Br J Radiol. 2005;78(926):161–3.
43. Zhang LJ, Yang GF, Qi J, Shen W. Renal artery aneurysm: diagnosis and surveillance with multidetector-row computed tomography. Acta Radiol. 2007;48(3):274–9.
44. Garg N, Pipinos II, Longo GM, Thorell WE, Lynch TG, Johanning JM. Detachable coils for repair of extraparenchymal renal artery aneurysms: an alternative to surgical therapy. Ann Vasc Surg. 2007;21(1):97–110.
45. Millard FC, Hemingway AP, Cumberland DC, Brown CB. Renal embolization for ablation of function in renal failure and hypertension. Postgrad Med J. 1989;65(768):729–34.
46. Keller FS, Coyle M, Rosch J, Dotter CT. Percutaneous renal ablation in patients with end-stage renal disease: alternative to surgical nephrectomy. Radiology. 1986;159(2):447–51.
47. Hahn ST, Park SH, Lee JM, Kim CY, Chang YS. Renal artery embolization controls intractable pain in a patient with polycystic kidney disease. Cardiovasc Intervent Radiol. 1999;22(5):422–4.
48. Harley JD, Shen FH, Carter SJ. Transcatheter infarction of a polycystic kidney for control of recurrent hemorrhage. AJR Am J Roentgenol. 1980;134(4):818–20.
49. Hom D, Eiley D, Lumerman JH, Siegel DN, Goldfischer ER, Smith AD. Complete renal embolization as an alternative to nephrectomy. J Urol. 1999;161(1):24–7.

Chapter 5
Splenic Artery Embolization for Non-surgical Splenectomy

Abstract Splenic artery embolization is a safe and effective alternative to surgical splenectomy, especially in patients who are poor surgical candidates due to associated co-morbidities.

It is an especially useful for the treatment of variceal bleeding due to hepatic cirrhosis. Splenic trauma can also be treated by embolization of the splenic artery. This treatment modality is especially useful where selective embolization is needed as when pseudoaneurysms of the splenic artery. These can be selectively embolized which enables tissue preservation without the need for splenectomy.

In clinical situations where hypersplenism prevents use of anti platelets for concomitant percutaneous coronary revascularization, splenic artery embolization is a safe alternative to surgical splenectomy prior to coronary revascularization, as in this scenario, a high grade coronary stenosis would be a relative contra-indication for surgical splenectomy.

Keywords Splenic trauma • Embolization • Splenectomy • Portal hypertension • Pseudoaneurysm

Introduction

In patients who have co-morbid conditions preventing splenectomy which itself carries significant morbidity and mortality, splenic artery embolization as a percutaneous procedure is a safe and effective therapeutic option. Splenic arterial interventions are performed to treat various clinical conditions, including abdominal trauma, hypersplenism, splenic arterial aneurysm, portal hypertension, and splenic neoplasm.

Here, we review the various clinical indications, techniques and complications of splenic artery embolization.

© Springer International Publishing Switzerland 2017

K. Varghese, S. Adhyapak, *Therapeutic Embolization*,
DOI 10.1007/978-3-319-42494-1_5

Anatomy of the Splenic Artery: Implications for Splenic Artery Embolization

The splenic artery supplies the spleen and some portions of the stomach and pancreas [1]. The splenic artery runs superior and anterior to the splenic vein, along the superior edge of the pancreas. Near the splenic hilum, the artery usually divides into superior and inferior terminal branches, and each branch further divides into four to six segmental intrasplenic branches. The superior terminal branches are usually longer than the inferior terminal branches and constitute the major arterial supply to the spleen. A superior polar artery usually arises from the distal splenic artery near the hilum, but it may originate from the superior terminal artery. The inferior polar artery usually gives rise to the left gastroepiploic artery, but the latter may also arise from the distal splenic or inferior terminal artery. The left gastroepiploic artery then runs along the greater curvature of the stomach. Numerous short gastric branches arise from the terminal splenic or left gastroepiploic artery to supply the gastric cardia and fundus.

The splenic artery has many branches that supply the pancreatic body and tail. The first large branch is the dorsal pancreatic artery, and the second large branch is the greater pancreatic artery (or arteria pancreatica magna), which arises from the middle segment of the splenic artery.

When embolization is planned, visualization of the pancreatic arteries is essential to reduce the risk of their unintended embolization (Fig. 5.1).

Splenic Trauma

The spleen is frequently injured in blunt abdominal trauma. Over the past few decades, the treatment of traumatic splenic injuries has moved substantially, from surgical towards nonsurgical management. The risk of fatal postsplenectomy sepsis or impaired resistance to certain infections has motivated the adoption of procedures that maximize splenic preservation [2].

A high range of failure rates (ranging from 2 to 52 %) with nonsurgical management, has resulted in a need for secondary splenectomy in some cases (3.4). This is especially so in cases of extensive splenic trauma. Computed tomography (CT) may be useful for detecting extravasation of contrast material–enhanced blood or pseudoaneurysm suggestive of active hemorrhage and for classifying splenic injury according to its severity. The risk of nonsurgical management failure was 44 % in patients with extensive splenic injury [3].

Indications for Splenic Artery Embolization

Surgical splenectomy is usually performed in patients who have traumatic injuries to the spleen and unstable hemodynamics, whereas splenic injuries in patients with stable hemodynamics are treated with nonsurgical management.

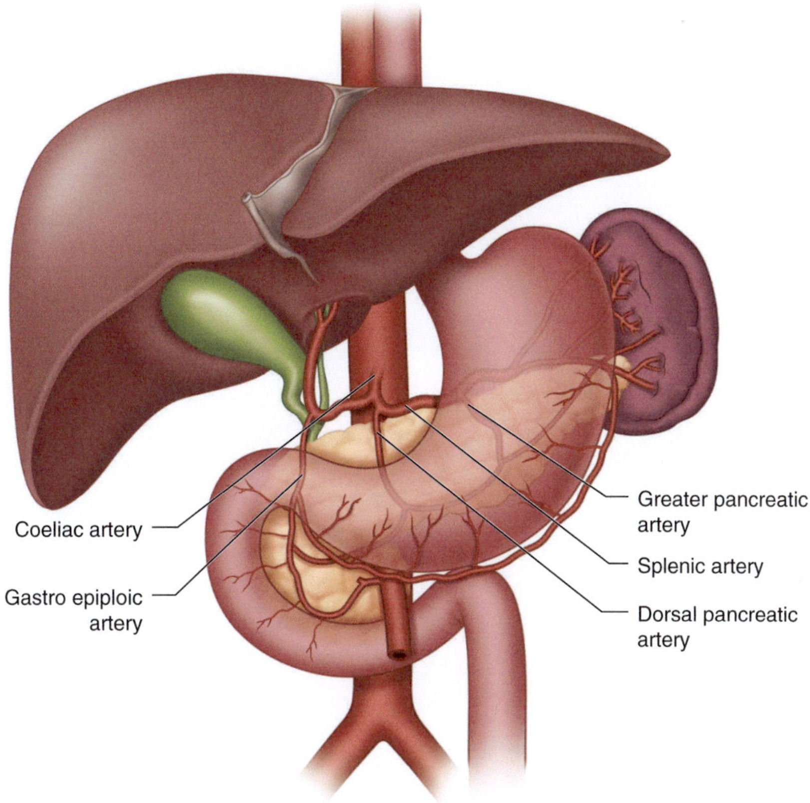

Fig. 5.1 Three-dimensional drawing of normal anatomy in the upper abdomen showing the main splenic artery and its branches

The most widely accepted indication for this procedure is evidence of arterial injury on CT scans. In cases of arterial injury, embolization is performed with microcoils as distally as possible, in a small arterial branch that supplies the segment in which extravasation, pseudoaneurysm, or abrupt termination is depicted, to preserve perfusion to the remaining splenic parenchyma. Patients with a high risk for secondary rupture of the spleen should undergo embolization with coils in a more proximal segment of the splenic artery to reduce the pressure in the splenic parenchyma and help the spleen to heal [4]. The placement of coils in a middle segment of the splenic artery allows reconstitution of the blood supply through collateral vessels, principally via the short gastric and gastroepiploic arteries, to the patent distal splenic, transgastric, and transpancreatic arteries. Proximal embolization performed exclusively with coils decreases volume of splenic arterial blood flow and thereby produces relative hypotension in the splenic bed, which allows the spleen to repair itself without infarction [5].

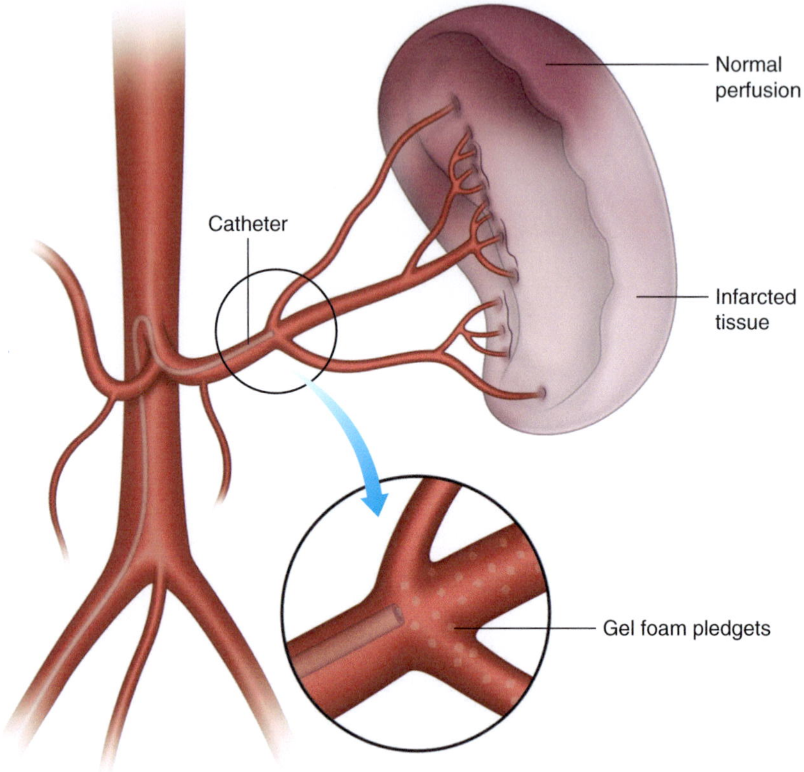

Fig. 5.2 Three-dimensional drawing of nonselective partial splenic arterial embolization with gelatin sponge pledgets shows patchy changes in perfusion (*brown areas*) throughout the splenic parenchyma

Technique of Splenic Artery Embolization

At angiography, frank extravasation is rare. More commonly, an arteriovenous fistula, pseudoaneurysm, or abrupt vessel truncation is seen.

A unique appearance characterized by punctate areas of parenchymal blush in the intrasplenic arteries may be observed and is usually indicates splenic contusion [6].

A patient whose hemodynamic condition becomes unstable during the procedure may require immediate proximal embolization of the splenic artery. Extensive injury involving multiple arterial branches usually requires proximal embolization of the splenic artery.

The decision to use a particular embolic agent depends on the ability to access the target vessel and on the nature of the lesion. When accessible, arteriovenous fistulas and pseudoaneurysms are treated with coils and/or gelatin sponges which are used to augment hemostasis. The incidence of segmental splenic infarction and intrasplenic air is increased with distal embolization [7] (Fig. 5.2). The presence of air in the spleen, unlike that in other organ systems, does not always indicate abscess formation.

Splenic abscess as a complication occurs in a small percentage of patients and may be successfully managed percutaneously or intraoperatively [7, 8]. Splenic salvage rates are similar whether embolization is performed in an artery segment distal or proximal to the splenic artery origin [9].

Results of Embolization

Haan et al. [10] analyzed the results of splenic arterial embolization in 40 patients in whom there was angiographic evidence of splenic vascular injury.

In 92 % of these 40 patients, nonsurgical salvage was successful; in 10 %, repeat angiography was required for suspected re-bleeding; and in half of these (5 %), a second embolization procedure was necessary. Bessoud et al. [11] studied all patients with splenic lacerations with evidence of extravasation on CT scans and stable hemodynamic status. The investigators in that study observed a 2.7 % failure rate in a group of 37 patients who underwent treatment with this technique, compared with a failure rate of 10 % for nonsurgical management in 30 patients. The group that underwent splenic arterial embolization had less morbidity, despite significantly higher CT grades of splenic trauma and a higher percentage of extravasation before intervention.

Hypersplenism

Surgical removal or transcatheter ablation of splenic parenchyma is often performed for the management of hypersplenism, a pathologic condition that is characterized by increased pooling or destruction of the corpuscular elements of the blood by the spleen [12]. Hypersplenism may be seen in many disorders, including cirrhosis with portal hypertension [13, 14]; hematologic abnormalities such as idiopathic thrombocytopenic purpura, thalassemia major, and hereditary spherocytosis. [15–18]; and diffuse splenic infiltration from primary malignancies such as leukemia and lymphoma [19, 20]. Signs of hypersplenism include splenomegaly, thrombocytopenia, leukopenia, and anemia, and symptoms may include abdominal discomfort, pain, respiratory distress, and early satiety [21, 22].

Here, total splenectomy may cause immunosuppression with susceptibility to encapsulated organism infections. Patients with co morbid conditions and severe cytopenia may benefit with partial splenic embolization. Many authors have advocated incomplete or partial splenic arterial embolization, in which a portion of the splenic parenchyma is left viable to preserve the spleen's immunologic function. Partial splenic arterial embolization has evolved after initial attempts to treat hypersplenism with proximal splenic arterial occlusion proved unsuccessful.

Treatment failures were attributed to abundant collateral circulation via short gastric and gastroepiploic arteries that reestablished the splenic blood supply around the occluded segment of the splenic artery. Although proximal arterial occlusion is ineffective for the management of hypersplenism, it is useful as a preoperative technique for reducing intraoperative blood loss in thrombocytopenic patients undergoing surgical splenectomy [23, 24].

The hematologic response and the severity of complications correlate with the amount of infracted splenic tissue. Splenic artery embolization resulting in infarction of more than 80 % of the splenic mass has been reported, but most interventionalists have attempted to achieve infarction in 60–70 % of the splenic mass [25, 26]. A lesser extent of infarction allows reduced sequestration and destruction of the blood elements, maintenance of the spleen's immunologic function, and preservation of antegrade flow in the splenic vein. However, complete splenic infarction may be beneficial immediately before splenectomy in patients who have severe thrombocytopenia and who will receive platelet transfusions during surgery.

Techniques of Partial Splenic Embolization

Partial splenic arterial embolization may be performed by two methods. With the first approach, selective partial embolization, a few distal branches of the splenic artery are selectively catheterized, and embolization is performed to achieve complete stasis in these branches while several other branches are left untreated (Fig. 5.2). Parenchymal phase angiograms may be used to estimate the volume of the remaining viable splenic tissue. Additional branches then may be catheterized, and embolization may be repeated, until the desired effect is achieved. With the second method, nonselective partial embolization, the working catheter tip is positioned more proximally in the main splenic artery but beyond the origin of major pancreatic branches and embolic particles are injected until the parenchymal blush is reduced. Contrast-enhanced CT may be used for follow-up examination.

The embolic agents most commonly used for splenic arterial embolization are gelatin sponge pledgets and polyvinyl alcohol particles. Coils have also been used for pre-operative embolization.

Due to the high incidence of associated morbidity with embolization of more than 80 % of splenic tissue, a more conservative approach may be prudent at initial embolization, which may be followed by a second embolization procedure if necessary.

Complications of Splenic Embolization

The use of total splenic infarction has been limited because of the high incidence and severity of complications such as splenic abscess, splenic rupture, septicemia, splenic vein thrombosis, and unremitting bronchopneumonia [27].

Several mechanisms may cause complications after complete splenic infarction: immunosuppression, anaerobic bacterial growth in the hypoxic tissue, percutaneous introduction of exogenous bacteria, and retrograde transport of enteric pathogens via a reversed portal flow.

In addition, patients may develop pleural effusions that require thoracentesis; paralytic ileus; pancreatitis due to nontarget embolization of the dorsal pancreatic or greater pancreatic artery; or postembolization syndrome, which consists of fever, leukocytosis, and abdominal pain.

Partial embolization has a lesser incidence of these complications.

Results of Partial Embolization

The use of partial splenic arterial embolization to manage variceal hemorrhage in patients with portal hypertension has been described in a limited number of reports [23, 28–31]. Embolization may be performed alone or in combination with other therapeutic interventions, such as endoscopic ligation [32, 33] or retrograde transvenous variceal obliteration [34]. The reduction of splenic volume results in a decrease in venous drainage and, thus, a reduction in portal venous flow and pressure.

Xu et al. [35] reported their experience with endoscopic variceal ligation and partial splenic arterial embolization in 41 patients in whom they evaluated the hemodynamic (blood flow rate and maximum flow velocity) effects of combination therapy. Esophageal varices and hypersplenism were well controlled, without recurrent hemorrhage (mean follow-up interval, 9.9 months), and there was a significant reduction in flow rate and maximum flow velocity in the main portal vein. Postembolization splenic abscess occurred in one patient, and another patient died of a pulmonary embolus. These results suggest a potential role for partial splenic arterial embolization in the spectrum of therapies used to manage morbid portal hypertension, especially in patients with advanced liver dysfunction and encephalopathy, conditions in which the use of a transjugular intrahepatic portosystemic shunt may not be viable.

Complications of partial splenic arterial embolization consisted mainly of fever, atelectasis, and abdominal pain, although two patients died as a result of more serious complications (severe hepatic insufficiency in one patient and complete splenic infarction with abscess, total portal vein thrombosis, and cardiac insufficiency in another patient). Thus, a standardized and graded partial embolization procedure is reasonably safe even in patients with advanced disease who are not candidates for surgery.

Splenic Artery Aneurysm

Splenic artery aneurysms are the most common visceral artery aneurysms, with a reported prevalence of 0.8 % at arteriography and 0.04–0.10 % at autopsy. Most aneurysms are small (<2 cm in diameter), saccular, and located at a bifurcation in a middle or distal segment of the splenic artery.

Splenic artery aneurysms are multiple in some, roughly 20 % of cases. Splenic artery aneurysms are found to have a predilection for multiparous women. Hormonal and hemodynamic alterations specific to pregnancy are likely contribute to intimal hyperplasia and fragmentation, which in turn may lead to aneurysm.

The prevalence of splenic artery aneurysm is substantially increased in patients with portal hypertension and is estimated at 7–20 % in patients with cirrhosis. Splenic artery pseudoaneurysm secondary to digestion of the arterial wall by proteolytic pancreatic enzymes may be seen in patients with pancreatitis. Other uncommon causes of splenic artery aneurysm include fibromuscular dysplasia, infection, and congenital anomalies.

Indications for treatment of splenic artery aneurysm or pseudoaneurysm include specific symptoms (e.g., epigastric pain, left upper quadrant pain, back pain), female sex and childbearing age, presence of portal hypertension, planned liver transplantation, a pseudoaneurysm of any size, and an aneurysm with a diameter of more than 2.5 cm.

Surgery for splenic artery aneurysms is associated with a mortality rate of approximately 1 %, but mortality is increased in patients with pancreatitis, in whom it is 16 % for those with aneurysms in the pancreatic head and 50 % for those with pancreatic body aneurysms.

Splenic artery aneurysms also may be treated with percutaneous interventional techniques such as transcatheter embolization, placement of a covered stent-graft to exclude the aneurysm in large aneurysms, or percutaneous injection of coils and/or thrombin.

Transcatheter embolization is associated with significantly lower morbidity and mortality than surgical procedures [36, 37]. Precise selection of the occlusion site is necessary to preserve collateral blood flow to the spleen via the gastric, omental, and pancreatic vessels.

Occlusion of the aneurysmal sac with embolic agents (most commonly with coils, detachable balloons or inert particles) and exclusion of the aneurysmal neck with the "sandwich" method are the recommended techniques for treating splenic artery aneurysms.

In large aneurysms [38, 39] placement of stent-graft across the aneurysmal neck to exclude the aneurysm, provides the benefit of preserving blood flow through the splenic artery. Flexible self-expanding stent-grafts can be delivered through small-bore introducer catheters (microcatheters) that can be manipulated within the tortuous splenic vasculature.

Possible complications include postembolization syndrome, transient elevation of pancreatic enzymes [40], splenic infarction, infection, abscess, and, rarely, rupture of a pseudoaneurysm. Follow-up imaging with CT or Doppler ultrasonography is recommended for assessment of the adequacy of treatment.

Portal Hypertension

The major sequelae of portal hypertension include variceal hemorrhage, hypersplenism, and hepatogenic ascites. A contributing factor to thrombocytopenia in patients with cirrhosis and portal hypertension is an increased platelet pool in the enlarged spleen [46]. The combination of varices and a low platelet count puts these patients at high risk for catastrophic hemorrhage.

Partial Splenic Embolization

The use of partial splenic arterial embolization to manage variceal hemorrhage in patients with portal hypertension has been described [23, 41–43]. Embolization may be performed alone or in combination with other therapeutic interventions, such as endoscopic ligation [44, 45] or retrograde transvenous variceal obliteration [52]. The reduction of splenic volume results in a decrease in venous drainage and, thus, a reduction in portal venous flow and pressure.

Liver Transplantation

Increased blood flow to the spleen as a result of decreased splenic arteriolar resistance is a common finding in patients with chronic liver disease and portal hypertension. Definitive treatment of liver failure with orthotopic liver transplantation can be complicated by the diversion of arterial blood flow away from the donor liver. Concurrent disease in the recipient, such as hepatitis or transplant rejection, can lead to an increase in hepatic arterial resistance, which results in the shunting of even more blood from the celiac axis toward the spleen. The triad of liver failure, reduced hepatic arterial perfusion, and increased blood flow in the splenic circulation after liver transplantation is called splenic artery steal syndrome.

Its clinical manifestations mimic the more common causes of graft failure, such as graft rejection or ischemia. In addition, splenic artery steal syndrome may manifest from a few hours to several weeks after surgery. Transplant surgeons must recognize this syndrome as a rare (estimated frequency, 3–4 %) but serious complication of liver transplantation [46].

Treatment of Splenic Artery Steal Syndrome

Surgical and endovascular approaches that have been proposed for treatment of splenic artery steal syndrome include surgical splenectomy, splenic artery ligation, creation of a new vascular conduit from the aorta to the hepatic artery, and splenic arterial embolization. Because liver transplant recipients are poor surgical candidates after transplantation, minimally invasive approaches to treating this syndrome are successful. Controversy exists, in the scarce literature on this subject, about whether or not repeat surgical ligation of the hepatic artery to the aorta or splenic arterial embolization should be considered the first-line therapy.

Uflacker et al. [49] reported their findings of splenic artery steal syndrome in a series of 11 patients after liver transplantation. The diagnosis was confirmed with celiac artery angiography, and therapeutic embolization was performed with coils in the middle segment of the splenic artery.

Immediate clinical improvement was noted in all patients. The authors reported only one procedure- related complication (hepatic artery thrombosis, which necessitated surgical repair). The authors noted that if hyperdynamic circulation to the spleen was observed intraoperatively, surgical anastomosis of the donor hepatic artery to the aorta should be performed to prevent splenic artery steal syndrome.

Splenic Neoplasia

Transarterial Splenic Irradiation

For years, splenic irradiation has been an effective treatment for lymphoma, leukemia, myelofibrosis, idiopathic thrombocytopenic purpura, and polycythemia vera with or without splenomegaly [42–44]. Although radiation therapy in solid organ malignancies has involved the use of external-beam radiation, the use of transarterial applications of irradiation, in patients with inoperable intrahepatic malignancy [45–47] is useful. The use of transarterial splenic irradiation with yttrium-90 microspheres has demonstrated beneficial clinical results with reduction of splenic volume and increase in platelet counts [48–50].

Combination Therapy

Another possibility for treatment of solid organ malignancies that has attracted recent interest is the combination of arterial embolization with therapeutic modalities such as radiofrequency ablation [51]. It is hypothesized that this therapy combination helps to increase the ablation zone by reducing the heat sink effect, which is the escape of thermal energy via moving blood.

Liu et al. [52] performed a study in 16 dogs to assess the feasibility and safety of radiofrequency ablation in the treatment of splenomegaly. Sixteen dogs were randomly divided into two groups, group 1 ($n=4$) and group 2 ($n=12$). Splenomegaly was induced with ligation of the splenic vein and its collateral branches in all dogs in both groups. After 3 weeks, radiofrequency ablation was performed in the spleen of the group 2 dogs. Complications of radiofrequency ablation were observed, CT was performed, the spleens were harvested, and the thermal lesions and histopathologic specimens from the spleen were examined. The authors observed segmental thermal lesions that had a hyperintense central zone of coagulative necrosis and a more extensive hypointense peripheral zone of infarction. The infarcted zone was absorbed and disappeared within 4–6 weeks after radiofrequency ablation, while the remaining spleen shrank.

The fundamental histopathologic changes caused by radiofrequency-induced heating included the creation of lesions with a central zone of coagulative necrosis and peripheral zone of thrombotic infarction, subsequent tissue absorption and fibrosis in the zone of thrombotic infarction, the occlusion of vessels in the remnant of viable spleen, the deposition of extensive fibrous protein, and the disappearance of congestive splenic sinusoid. No complication or death occurred in either group. Liu and colleagues concluded that radiofrequency ablation of the spleen is feasible and safe. Although the results achieved in the two groups were similar, the use of partial splenic arterial embolization before radiofrequency ablation may help to improve both the experimental and the clinical results of ablation.

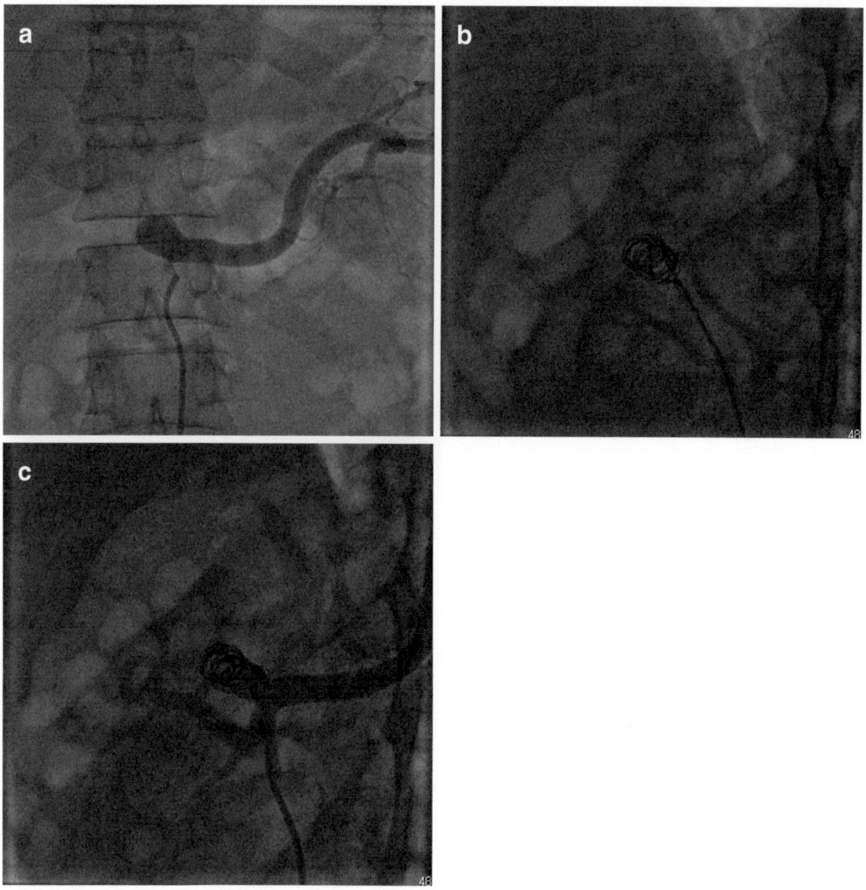

Fig. 5.3 (**a**) Splenic angiogram demonstrating a pseudo aneurysm, which was embolised (**b**) using multiple coils, and (**c**) post coil embolization angiogram showing occlusion of the pseudoaneurysm

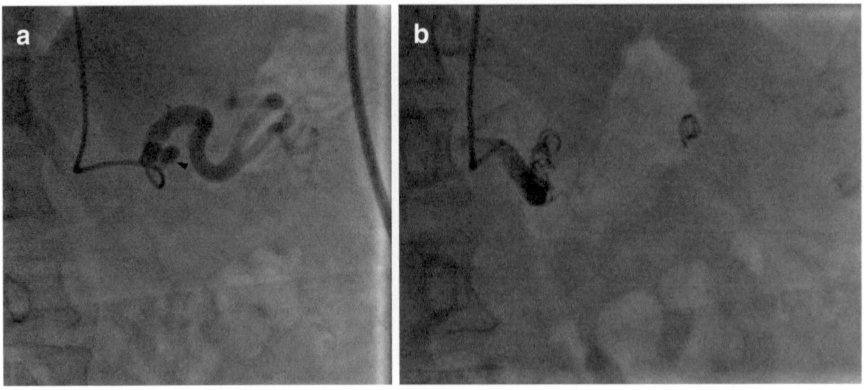

Fig. 5.4 (**a**, **b**) Splenic angiogram done through brachial arterial access demonstrating a pseudoaneurysm and the post- embolization angiogram showing occlusion

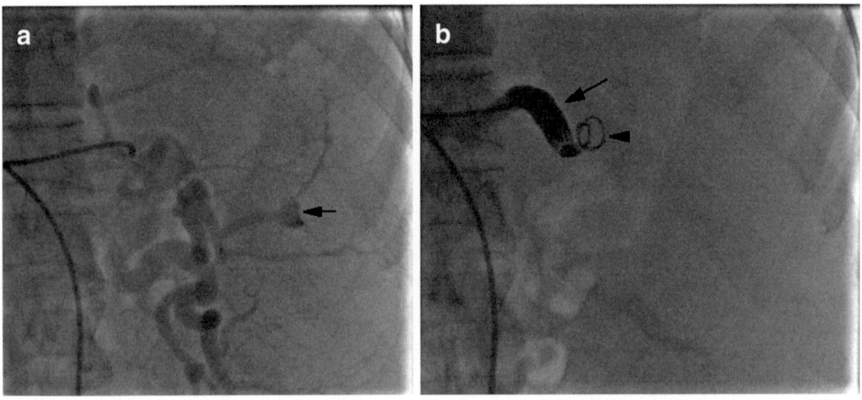

Fig. 5.5 (**a**) Splenic angiogram demonstrating a pseudo aneurysm (*black arrow*) and post embolization angiogram (**b**) showing occlusion of the splenic artery (*arrow*) using a coil (*arrowhead*)

Given the encouraging results described, further investigation of combination therapies for splenomegaly and primary and secondary splenic malignancies is needed.

Our Experience

We have performed splenic artery embolizations for traumatic pseudoaneurysms in two patients, pseudoaneurysms associated with pancreatitis in five patients (Figs. 5.3, 5.4, and 5.5) and for idiopathic thrombocytopenic purpura in one patient in whom surgical splenectomy was high risk due to a high grade stenosis in the left anterior descending coronary artery. He needed a splenic embolization prior to coronary stenting as a staged procedure after improvements in platelet count after splenic embolization [53].

Conclusions

Splenic arterial interventions may be used to treat a wide range of pathologic entities.

As the indications for splenic arterial interventions increase, a thorough knowledge of the common techniques and their potential pitfalls and complications will be necessary.

References

1. Kadir S, Lundell C, Saeed M. Celiac, superior and inferior mesenteric arteries. In: Kadir S, editor. Atlas of normal and variant angiographic anatomy. Philadelphia: Saunders; 1991. p. 204–37.
2. Cullingford GL, Watkins DN, Watts AD, Mallon DF. Severe late postsplenectomy infection. Br J Surg. 1991;78:716–21.
3. Velmahos GC, Toutouzas KG, Radin R, Chan L, Demetriades D. Nonoperative treatment of blunt injury to solid abdominal organs. Arch Surg. 2003;138:844–51.
4. Albrecht RM, Schermer CR, Morris A. Nonoperative management of blunt splenic injuries: factors influencing success in age _55 years. Am Surg. 2002;68:227–30.
5. Sclafani SJ, Shaftan GW, Scalea TM, et al. Nonoperative salvage of computed tomography-diagnosed splenic injuries: utilization of angiography for triage and embolization for hemostasis. J Trauma. 1995;39:818–25.
6. Link DP, Seibert JA, Gould J, Lantz BM. On-line monitoring of sequential blood flow reduction during splenic embolization. Acta Radiol. 1989;30:101–3.
7. Levy JM, Wasserman PI, Weiland DE. Nonsuppurative gas formation in the spleen after transcatheter splenic infarction. Radiology. 1981;139:375–6.
8. Killeen KL, Shanmuganathan K, Boyd-Kranis R, Scalea TM, Mirvis SE. CT findings after embolization for blunt splenic trauma. J Vasc Interv Radiol. 2001;12:209–14.
9. Haan J, Bochicchio G, Kramer M, Scalea T. Air following splenic embolization: infection or incidental finding? Am Surg. 2003;69:1036–9.
10. Haan JM, Biffl W, Knudson MM, et al. Splenic embolization revisited: a multicenter review. J Trauma. 2004;56:542–7.
11. Kramer M, Scalea TM. Admission angiography for blunt splenic injury: advantages and pitfalls. J Trauma. 2001;51:1161–5.
12. Bessoud B, Denys A. Main splenic artery embolization using coils in blunt splenic injuries: effects on the intrasplenic blood pressure. Eur Radiol. 2004;14:1718–9.
13. Peck-Radosavljevic M. Hypersplenism. Eur J Gastroenterol Hepatol. 2001;13:317–23.
14. Sangro B, Bilbao I, Herrero I, et al. Partial splenic embolization for the treatment of hypersplenism in cirrhosis. Hepatology. 1993;18:309–14.
15. Romano M, Giojelli A, Capuano G, Pomponi D, Salvatore M. Partial splenic embolization in patients with idiopathic portal hypertension. Eur J Radiol. 2004;49:268–73.
16. Stanley P, Chen TC. Partial embolization of the spleen in patients with thalassemia. J Vasc Interv Radiol. 1995;6:137–42.

17. Kimura F, Ito H, Shimizu H, et al. Partial splenic embolization for the treatment of hereditary spherocytosis. AJR Am J Roentgenol. 2003;181:1021–4.
18. Kumar S, Diehn FE, Gertz MA, Tefferi A. Splenectomy for immune thrombocytopenic purpura: long-term results and treatment of postsplenectomy relapses. Ann Hematol. 2002;81:312–9.
19. Miyazaki M, Itoh H, Kaiho T, et al. Partial splenic embolization for the treatment of chronic idiopathic thrombocytopenic purpura. AJR Am J Roentgenol. 1994;163:123–6.
20. Athale UH, Kaste SC, Bodner SM, Ribeiro RC. Splenic rupture in children with hematologic malignancies. Cancer. 2000;88:480–90.
21. Gardner RV, Warrier RP, Loe W, Ward K, Haymon M, Craver R. Splenic artery embolization as emergency treatment of splenic rupture in a child with T-cell acute lymphocytic leukemia having t(8;14) translocation. Med Pediatr Oncol. 2003;41:492–3.
22. Pringle KC, Spigos DG, Tan WS, et al. Partial splenic embolization in the management of thalassemia major. J Pediatr Surg. 1982;17:884–91.
23. Jonasson O, Spigos DG, Mozes MF. Partial splenic embolization: experience in 136 patients. World J Surg. 1985;9:461–7.
24. Poulin EC, Mamazza J, Schlachta CM. Splenic artery embolization before laparoscopic splenectomy: an update. Surg Endosc. 1998;12:870–5.
25. Iwase K, Higaki J, Mikata S, et al. Laparoscopically assisted splenectomy following preoperative splenic artery embolization using contour emboli for myelofibrosis with massive splenomegaly. Surg Laparosc Endosc Percutan Tech. 1999;9:197–202.
26. Mozes MF, Spigos DG, Pollak R, et al. Partial splenic embolization, an alternative to splenectomy: results of a prospective, randomized study. Surgery. 1984;96:694–702.
27. Kumpe DA, Rumack CM, Pretorius DH, Stoecker TJ, Stellin GP. Partial splenic embolization in children with hypersplenism. Radiology. 1985;155:357–62.
28. Fukuda T, Yoshikawa T. Interventional radiologic treatment for idiopathic portal hypertension. Cardiovasc Intervent Radiol. 1999;22:311–4.
29. Shimizu T, Onda M, Tajiri T, et al. Bleeding portal- hypertensive gastropathy managed successfully by partial splenic embolization. Hepatogastroenterology. 2002;49:947–9.
30. Sato T, Yamazaki K, Toyota J, Karino Y, Ohmura T, Suga T. Gastric varices with splenic vein occlusion treated by splenic arterial embolization. J Gastroenterol. 2000;35:290–5.
31. Xu RY, Liu B, Lin N. Therapeutic effects of endoscopic variceal ligation combined with partial splenic embolization for portal hypertension. World J Gastroenterol. 2004;10:1072–4.
32. Taniai N, Onda M, Tajiri T, Toba M, Yoshida H. Endoscopic variceal ligation (EVL) combined with partial splenic embolization (PSE). Hepatogastroenterology. 1999;46:2849–53.
33. Chikamori F, Kuniyoshi N, Kawashima T, Shibuya S, Takase Y. Combination treatment of partial splenic embolization, endoscopic embolization and transjugular retrograde obliteration for complicated gastroesophageal varices. Hepatogastroenterology. 2004;51:1506–9.
34. Palsson B, Hallen M, Forsberg AM, Alwmark A. Partial splenic embolization: long-term outcome. Langenbecks Arch Surg. 2003;387:421–6.
35. McDermott VG, Shlansky-Goldberg R, Cope C. Endovascular management of splenic artery aneurysms and pseudoaneurysms. Cardiovasc Intervent Radiol. 1994;17:179–84.
36. Guillon R, Garcier JM, Abergel A, et al. Management of splenic artery aneurysms and false aneurysms with endovascular treatment in 12 patients. Cardiovasc Intervent Radiol. 2003;26:256–60.
37. Arepally A, Dagli M, Hofmann LV, Kim HS, Cooper M, Klein A. Treatment of splenic artery aneurysm with use of a stent-graft. J Vasc Interv Radiol. 2002;13:631–3.
38. Brountzos EN, Vagenas K, Apostolopoulou SC, Panagiotou I, Lymberopoulou D, Kelekis DA. Pancreatitis-associated splenic artery pseudoaneurysm: endovascular treatment with self-expandable stent-grafts. Cardiovasc Intervent Radiol. 2003;26:88–91.
39. De Carlis L, Sansalone CV, Rondinara GF, et al. Splenic artery steal syndrome after orthotopic liver transplantation: diagnosis and treatment. Transplant Proc. 1993;25:2594–6.
40. Uflacker R, Selby JB, Chavin K, Rogers J, Baliga P. Transcatheter splenic artery occlusion for treatment of splenic artery steal syndrome after orthotopic liver transplantation. Cardiovasc Intervent Radiol. 2002;25:300–6.

41. Galbraith PR. The mechanism of action of splenic irradiation in chronic myelogenous leukemia. Can Med Assoc J. 1967;96:1636–41.
42. Abrams RA, Liu PJ, Ambinder RF, et al. Hodgkin and non-Hodgkin lymphoma: local-regional radiation therapy after bone marrow transplantation. Radiology. 1997;203:865–70.
43. Elliott MA, Chen MG, Silverstein MN, Tefferi A. Splenic irradiation for symptomatic splenomegaly associated with myelofibrosis with myeloid metaplasia. Br J Haematol. 1998;103:505–11.
44. Schratter-Sehn AU, Cerveny M, Simmel H, Schlogl E, Schratter A. Short-time splenic irradiation for splenomegaly. Onkologie. 2003;26:21–4.
45. McFarland JT, Kuzma C, Millard FE, Johnstone PA. Palliative irradiation of the spleen. Am J Clin Oncol. 2003;26:178–83.
46. Herba MJ, Thirlwell MP. Radioembolization for hepatic metastases. Semin Oncol. 2002;29:152–9.
47. Salem R, Lewandowski R, Roberts C, et al. Use of yttrium-90 glass microspheres (TheraSphere) for the treatment of unresectable hepatocellular carcinoma in patients with portal vein thrombosis. J Vasc Interv Radiol. 2004;15:335–45.
48. Salem R, Thurston KG, Carr BI, Goin JE, Geschwind JF. Yttrium-90 microspheres: radiation therapy for unresectable liver cancer. J Vasc Interv Radiol. 2002;13(9 pt 2):S223–9.
49. Ariel IM, Padula G. Irradiation of the spleen by the intra-arterial administration of 90 yttrium microspheres in patients with malignant lymphoma: a preliminary report. Cancer. 1973;31:90–6.
50. Becker CD, Rosler H, Biasiutti FD, Baer HU. Congestive hypersplenism: treatment by means of radioembolization of the spleen with Y-90. Radiology. 1995;195:183–6.
51. Koda M, Ueki M, Maeda Y, et al. The influence on liver parenchymal function and complications of radiofrequency ablation or the combination with transcatheter arterial embolization for hepatocellular carcinoma. Hepatol Res. 2004;29:18–23.
52. Liu QD, Ma KS, He ZP, Ding J, Huang XQ, Dong JH. Experimental study on the feasibility and safety of radiofrequency ablation for secondary splenomagely and hypersplenism. World J Gastroenterol. 2003;9:813–7.
53. Varghese K, Viegas M, Adhyapak SM. A therapeutic dilemma – coronary artery stenting in the setting of thrombocytopaenia. Heart Lung Circ. 2015;24:e214–6.

Chapter 6
Uterine Artery Embolization for Bleeding due to Fibroids

Abstract Fibroids are benign tumors of the uterus causing excessive bleeding which have hitherto been subjected to surgical excision called myectomy. When unresectable, hysterectomy has been performed as a definitive therapy. An alternative minimally invasive procedure which is increasingly preferred as the treatment of choice is uterine artery embolization. A thorough knowledge of the vascular anatomy and technical expertise is required for successful embolization. The technical pitfalls require careful consideration to prevent procedural complications. This procedure has been safely applied even to large fibroids with successful results and minimal complications. Recurrence rates are low with restoration of blood flow to the uterus through collaterals from the ovarian and epigastric arteries. This procedure has also been tried with success to prevent post-partum bleeding after delivery with no maternal or fetal complications.

Keywords Uterine artery • Bleeding • Fibroid • Leiyomyoma • Carcinoma • Pudendal artery

Vascular Anatomy of the Female Genital Tract

With the expanding indications for vascular embolization of the female genital tract, it is vital to delineate the normal vascular anatomy and its variations [1]. This is necessary for safe embolization procedures and prevention of non-targeted embolization. The indications for uterine artery embolization range from fibroids, postpartum hemorrhage, neoplasms, vascular malformations associated with neoplasms and pelvic trauma.

The internal iliac artery terminated into two main stems, one anterior and one posterior, in 77 % of cases (Fig. 6.1). Other modes of division of the internal iliac artery were three stems in 14 %, four or more stems in 3 %, and one main stem in 4 % of cases. In all cases, the posterior trunk gave rise to the iliolumbar, the lateral sacral, and the superior gluteal arteries. The superior gluteal artery was invariably the terminal branch. The anterior division was not as well defined as the posterior stem. The origin of the uterine artery may not be usually visible on anteroposterior views. Contralateral anterior oblique is usually the best projection to visualize the

© Springer International Publishing Switzerland 2017

K. Varghese, S. Adhyapak, *Therapeutic Embolization*,
DOI 10.1007/978-3-319-42494-1_6

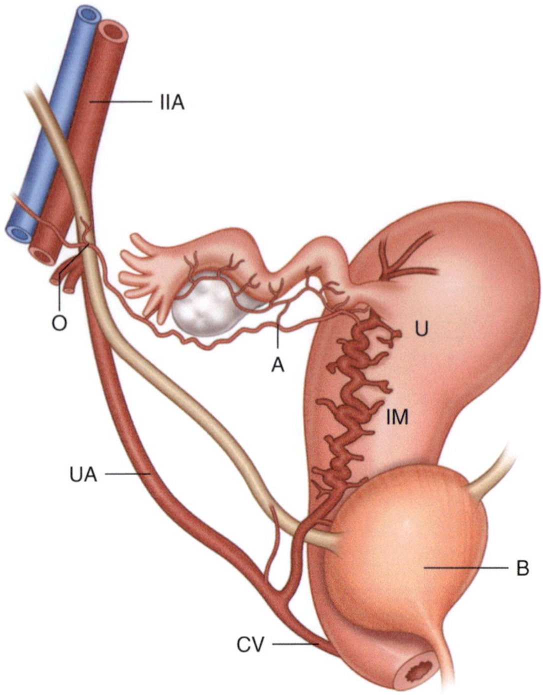

Fig. 6.1 Anatomic drawing of normal vascularization of uterus and adnexa shows internal iliac artery (*IIA*); ovarian artery (*0*) originating from abdominal aorta (not shown); uterine artery (*UA*); uterus (*U*); intramural branches (*IM*); bladder (*B*); and cervicovaginal artery (*CV*). *A* anastomoses between uterine and ovarian arteries

uterine artery when the uterine artery arises from the anterior division of the internal iliac artery (Fig. 6.2).

When the uterine artery originates from one, three, or four stems, ipsilateral anterior oblique may be the best projection for its visualization. The width of the uterine artery is subject to great variation. It varies between 2 and 5 mm. The uterine artery has a characteristic U-shaped course which consists of a parietal or descending segment running downward and medially a transversal ligament segment coursing medially, the uterine arch part, and the marginal or ascending segment running along the side of the uterus.

At the superior angle of the uterus, the artery penetrates into the broad ligament and divides into its terminal branches-tubal and ovarian-creating anastomoses with the ovarian artery branches.

Branches of the Uterine Artery

The cervicovaginal artery usually arises from the arch. When the utetine artery originates from the internal iliac artery, the cervico-vaginal branch may not be seen because of its small size. Intramural branches arising along the side of the uterus (also called arcuate arteries).

The terminal branches of the arcuate arteries were anastomose with those of the contralateral side.

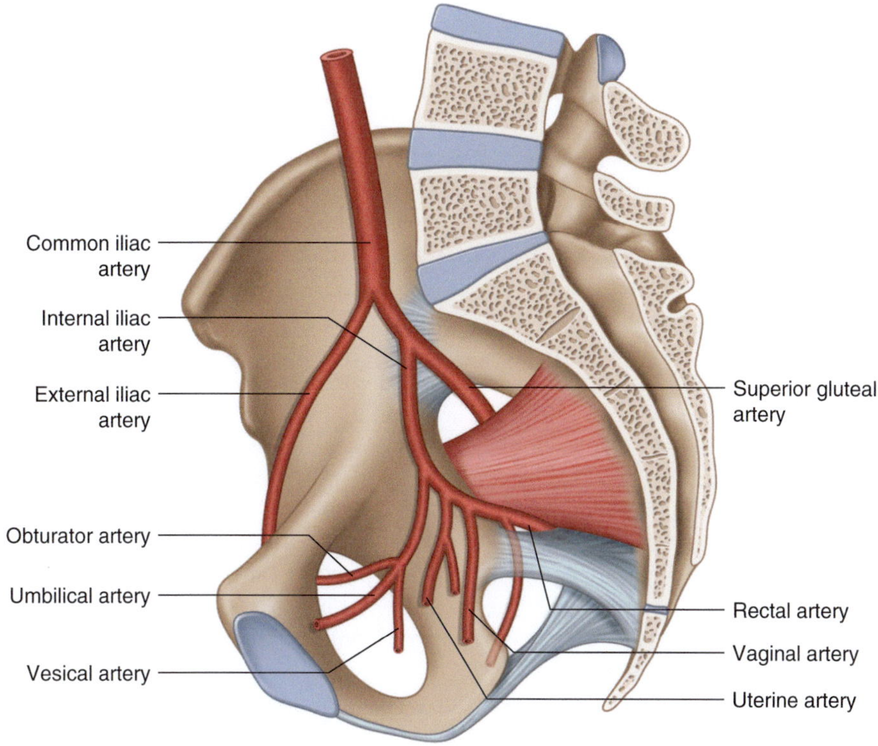

Fig. 6.2 Anatomic drawing shows lateral view of division of female internal iliac artery into two main stems. Note that uterine artery is branch of anterior division of internal iliac artery. Piriformis muscle (*orange*), sacrospinal ligament (*light green*), and sacrotuberal ligament (*dark green*) are also portrayed

Ovarian Artery

The ovarian artery arises anterolaterally from the abdominal aorta below the renal artery, at the level of the second lumbar vertebral body. The ovarian artery has a characteristic sinuous course. This artery anastomoses with the uterine artery.

Transverse anastomoses between the right and left uterine arteries is the usual pattern. Uterine arteries can anastomose with the ovarian arteries. Sometimes the round ligament artery which is a branch of the proximal epigastric artery can anastomose with the uterine artery.

The vaginal artery arises from the anterior division of the internal iliac artery just below the uterine artery. It usually arises from a common trunk formed with the uterine artery. The vesical artery, arises from the anterior division of the internal iliac artery usually above the uterine artery.

It takes a downward medial course to reach the lateral part of the bladder and gives off three terminal branches, which are easily identified when the bladder is full on angiography.

Anatomical Guides for Uterine Artery Embolization

The anatomy of the internal iliac artery is variable as it runs a variable course. The internal iliac artery terminates at the upper limit of the greater sciatic notch into two main stems, one anterior and one posterior, in most patients. The posterior division must be preserved during the embolization of the anterior branches of the internal iliac artery. The anterior division of the internal iliac artery is subject to numerous variations. During angiographic procedures, identification of these anterior branches, especially the parietal ones, is facilitated if bony landmarks and superselective catheterization may be required. Right and left symmetry of the branching pattern of the internal iliac artery is seen in most patients. The best projection to identify the origin of the uterine artery is the contralateral anterior oblique with 20^0–30^0 inclination. The width of the artery is subject to great variation; enlargement being common in pregnant patients and those with leiomyoma.

In the midline, the terminal parts of arcuate branches of the uterine artery anastomose with those of the contralateral side.

The paired ovarian arteries arise from the anterolateral abdominal aorta below the renal arteries. Although the uterine artery provides the dominant blood flow to the uterus, the ovarian artery is frequently involved in pathologic hypervascularized processes.

Each ovarian artery usually anastomoses with the corresponding terminal branches of the uterine artery.

The round ligament artery plays a minor role in physiologic conditions. This branch, which arises either from the inferior epigastric artery or from the external iliac artery, may anastomose with the uterine artery and become responsible for persistent bleeding after hysterectomy.

The vesical artery arises from the anterior division of the internal iliac artery, sometimes from a common trunk with the uterine artery. It has three vesical branches that supply 80 % of the blood flow to the bladder. Special care should be taken during uterine embolotherapy to avoid bladder necrosis by identifying these branches.

Identification of all branches of the internal iliac artery is necessary to avoid untargetted embolization. To perform safer embolization, the catheter should be carefully placed into the descending segment of the uterine artery. Similarly, failure of superselective catheterization of the uterine artery may lead to unilateral embolization and lack of therapeutic effect. Also, use of a hydrophilic polymer-coated 0.032-in. (rather than 0.035-in.) guidewire can prevent vasospasm of the uterine artery.

Indications for Uterine Artery Embolization

Uterine Fibroids

Uterine artery embolization was first introduced in 1995 as a treatment option for uterine fibroids [2]. An early analysis of a prospective registry with 3160 patients had a 5.5 % incidence of major complications at 30 days with a 0.1 % incidence of hysterectomy.

A randomized control trial was done comparing the outcomes of uterine artery embolization and hysterectomy, with a 1 year study period. Both uterine arteries were embolized using material of 500–710 μm diameter. The quality of life scores were assessed at 12 months and were similar in both groups, except that there was greater improvement in quality of life at 1 month in the embolization group.

Minor Complications

Minor complications were usually related to the postembolization syndrome in 52 %, which included pyrexia, pain, and elevated inflammatory markers and to minor infections in 25 % in the surgical group.

Major Complications

There were 16 major adverse events (15 %) in the embolization group, as compared with 10 (20 %) in the surgical group during a median follow-up of 32 months. When these were analysed according to the timing of their occurrence, 8 of the 10 major adverse events in the surgical group occurred during the hospital stay, whereas 15 of the 16 events in the embolization group occurred after discharge from the hospital.

Treatment Failures

Twenty-one patients (20 %) in the embolization group required an additional invasive procedure (hysterectomy or repeated uterine-artery embolization) for continued or recurrent symptoms, 10 during the first 12 months of follow-up (2 of which were due to technical failures) and 11 subsequently.

In the surgical group, there was one conversion of myomectomy to hysterectomy at the time of the primary procedure.

A cost minimization analysis was done which analysis showed that at 1 year, embolization was more cost-effective than surgery.

Situations of Large Fibroid Burden

In patients with large fibroids of >8–10 cm and or a uterine volume of >700 ML, uterine artery embolization is considered risky by some Interventionalists due to complications of such as unbearable pain, infection, septic uterine necrosis, and lethal sepsis. Uterine fibroid infarction rates were targeted to be atleast 80 % in most studies. A long term follow-up study (>5 years) of uterine artery embolization in this group was done, with achievement of infarction rates of <80 % in most of the patients labeled as inadequate infarction [3]. Some women developed temporary amenorrhoea while some developed permanent amenorrhoea. Fibroid expulsion and fibroid sloughing with vaginal discharge occurred in a minority. Post-procedure pain was rare as was the low occurrence of urogenital infection requiring antibiotics.

None developed post-embolization syndrome. In 11 % of patients there was need for a second embolization due to revascularization of the fibroid through the ovarian artery and inferior epigastric artery. The need for hysterectomy arose in 8 % of patients during follow-up. A quality of life questionnaire showed good clinical improvements at long term. This study demonstrates that uterine artery embolization procedure is safe and has good clinical outcomes even in cases of large fibroid burden. The risks of complications are less than predicted.

Long-term follow-up of patients who have undergone uterine artery embolization for leiomyoma at 2 years has proven its clinical efficacy [Leiomyoma]. Uterine leiomyoma is a benign and well-defined tumor of the myometrium that can have a submucosal, interstitial, or subserosal location.

It is surrounded by peripheral arteries from which centripetal arteries reach the core of the lesion. Uterine arteries are usually enlarged to supply these hypervascular networks and can easily be cannulated using a 4- or 5-French catheter. Catheterization of uterine arteries may be performed via the anterior trunks of the hypogastric arteries using a uni- or bilateral femoral artery approach. The single femoral artery approach is adequate to cannulate the contra-lateral and then ipsilateral uterine arteries. In order to avoid arterial vasospasm, some Interventionalists recommend ceasing hormone therapy such as gonadotrophin-releasing hormone analogs several weeks before treatment. Because superselective catheterization of the small arteries supplying leiomyomas is not possible, embolization with polymerizing liquid emboli is contraindicated. Free flow injection of calibrated particles (polyvinyl alcohol) is therefore preferred and can be performed in both uterine arteries to induce devascularization of leiomyomas.

About 40–50 % reduction in the size of leiomyoma was observed on sonographic examination at follow-up. Pain relief was seen in almost all patients immediately after the procedure and none had any ischemic complications with a recurrence in about 2 % requiring repeat embolization. Recurrence following myectomy was nearly 25 % which required hysterectomy. Post-procedural amenorrhoea was seen in 1 % and was found to be related to menopause and not to the procedure itself.

Usage Patterns of Uterine Artery Embolization (UAE)

The Cochrane review from 2006 cited that UAE resulted in the same patient satisfaction rate as surgery (myomectomy or hysterectomy) [4]. The length of hospital stay was lesser after UFE, and the return to daily activities was faster. Because UAE seemed to result in a higher minor complication rate and more unscheduled visits and readmission rates, the statement was made that additional focus on long-term follow-up was necessary to determine its real impact.

Although UAE as an alternative treatment for hysterectomy or myomectomy is widespread in Europe, its impact on the management of patients with symptomatic fibroid seemed, according to the overall numbers of UAE procedures, disappointing.

In countries like India, this is more so due to lack of adequate dissemination of information about the safety and efficacy of the procedure as an effective alternative to surgical myectomy/hysterectomy for symptomatic uterine fibroids.

Rare Indications for UAE

Abnormal Placentation

Abnormal placentation, which broadly comprises placenta previa, accreta, increta, and percreta, is a leading cause of massive peripartum hemorrhage. It frequently leads to emergency hysterectomies, surgical manipulation of organs adjacent to the uterus (ureter and bladder), respiratory distress syndrome, kidney failure, and even death. Blood loss in cesarean sections among patients with placental accreta can vary from 3,000 to 5,000 mL.

A hybrid procedure of UAE and caesarian section was done in 12 patients to assess the safety and efficacy of the procedure [5]. In an operating theatre fitted with a mobile C-Arm and DSA angiography, the bilateral uterine arteries were cannulated. Then, the infant was delivered, umbilical cord was clamped and any bleeding vessels were clamped, vagina was packed with the placenta in situ. Both uterine arteries were embolized using Gelfoam until there was flow cessation. There was no fetal or maternal mortality. Two patients needed hysterectomy, as both had extreme placenta previa. The average radiation dose was 91.79 mGy (range 30.2–71), and the average dose area product was 2.37 mGym2 (range 0.849–4.09).

The average blood loss during the surgical procedure of all 12 cases was 1,391 mL (range 600–3,600), and the average urinary amount was 358 mL (range 200–500). None had complications of infection or hemorrhage. The volume of vaginal bleeding was approximately 80 mL (range 20–150). The mean postoperative hospitalization time was 8.75 days (range 7–10).

In 10 of 12 patients, the uterus was successfully preserved with complete placental removal after prophylactic bilateral UAE. Blood loss was minimal and there was no post-operative infection. There was no incidence of post-embolization syndrome. The radiation dose was also minimal. This was mainly due to unilateral uterine artery cannulation. According to the National Council on Radiation Protection and Measurements, the risk to an infant from fluoroscopy dosage is increased significantly when the radiation exposure exceeds 150 mGy [6, 7].

However, at doses of \50 mGy, the risk of radiation induced abnormality is considered negligible compared with baseline risks for all developmental abnormalities, e.g., 1 % for mental retardation and 3 % for spontaneous birth defects [6, 8].

The risk of increased surgery time and patient morbidity and mortality seen in earlier studies which required shifting of the patients to the operation theatre after uterine artery cannulation in the catheterization laboratory was avoided as the portable C –Arm and DSA angiography was available in the operation theatre. This also facilitated a second embolization procedure if required.

Complications of UAE

The incidence of major complications has been reported as 4 % and minor complications as 23 % [9]. The acute complications are generally related to those of vascular access, especially where vascular access is associated with sutures. These complications include arterial dissection, pseudoaneurysm, lower extremity emboli, puncture site hematoma, contrast allergy, contrast nephropathy, nerve injury, and infection.

An increased incidence was seen with use of suture mediated devices for access closure than with manual compression. A very rare complication was thromboembolic manifestations including deep vein thrombosis and pulmonary thromboembolism.

Infections like endometritis and sepsis are rare complications associated with UFE. Delayed superinfection of necrotic, dominant fibroids has been described weeks to months after UFE in case reports, occasionally resulting in sepsis and requiring myomectomy or hysterectomy.

Uterine necrosis is a rare, major complication associated with UFE that if not aggressively treated can result in sepsis and death. At least three deaths are documented in the literature associated with UFE.

Non-target embolization in one patient resulted in labial necrosis associated with ovarian failure and unilateral deep buttock pain.

Expulsion or discharge of small tissue fragments and necrotic material is a common minor complication of UFE, occurring in 2.5 % of patients. Chronic vaginal discharge following UFE often results when a small communication forms between an infarcted, superficial fibroid and the endometrial cavity.

Amenorrhea, both transient and permanent, has been reported as a complication associated with UFE. Permanent amenorrhea may result from nontarget embolization of the ovaries with resulting ovarian dysfunction, or secondary to endometrial atrophy.

Treatment Failure

Treatment Failure was defined as "subsequent hysterectomy, definitive myomectomy, repeat embolization, or failure of symptom improvement at the patient's final follow-up."

Possible causes of failure of treatment include incomplete embolization, arterial spasm, recanalization of the arteries, prominent nonuterine artery collateral supply, and persistent effects of gonadotropin agonists.

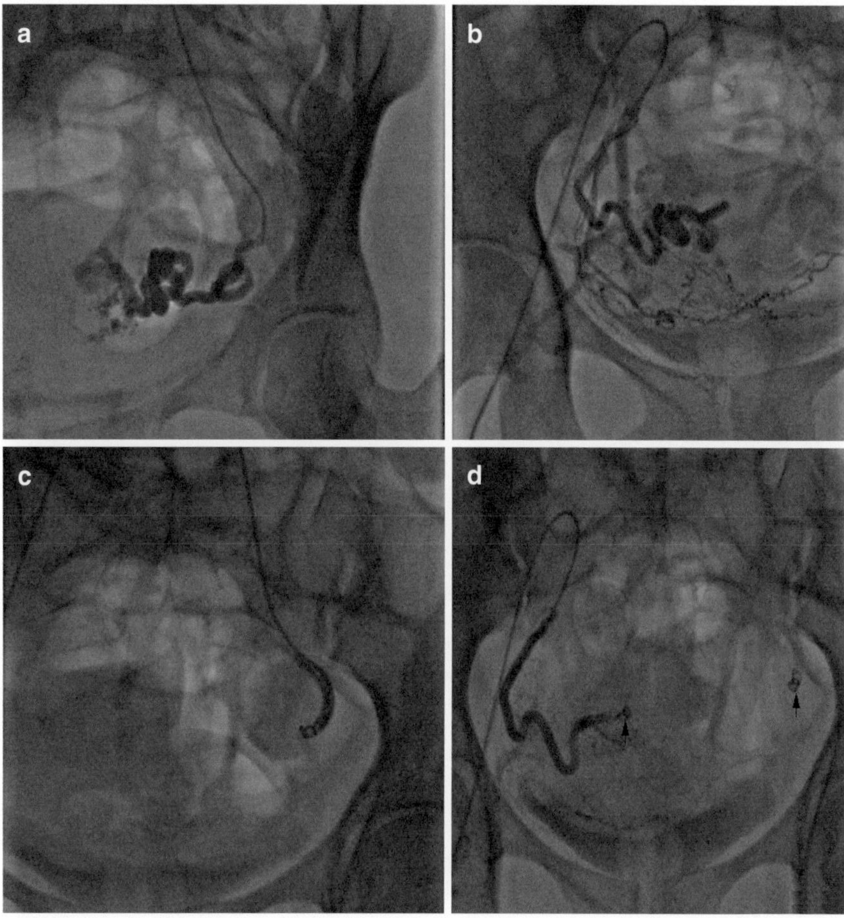

Fig. 6.3 (**a**–**c**) Uterine artery embolization in a patient with menorrhagia and AVM. Feeding arteries from the left internal iliac artery (**a**) and right internal iliac artery (**b**) were successfully embolised (**c**) and (**d**) using coils (*arrows*)

Subsequent Pregnancies

There was a high incidence of caesarian sections in pregnancies following UAE. Persistant necrotic material was a contra-indication for subsequent pregnancies.

Our Experience

We have performed 12 UAE procedures for fibroids with excessive bleeding. We have had a 92.7 % success rate with one patient requiring hysterectomy (8.3 %) (Figs. 6.3a–d).

Conclusion

UAE is a safe and clinically effective minimally invasive therapy for uterine fibroids and is an alternative to hysterectomy even in large fibroids. It can also be applied in cases of abnormal placentation during caesarian section with caution. There is a need for widespread awareness about this procedure as a therapy for fibroids.

References

1. Pelage J-P, Le Dref O, Soyer P, Jacob D, KardaChe M, Dahan H, Lassau J-P, Rymer R. Arterial anatomy of the female genital tract: variations and relevance to transcatheter embolization of the uterus. Am J Radiol. 1999;172:989–94.
2. The Writing Committee of the Randomized Trial of Embolization versus Surgical Treatment for Fibroids consisted of Richard D. Edwards, M.B., Ch.B., and Jonathan G. Moss, M.B., Ch.B., Gartnavel Hospital; Mary Ann Lumsden, M.D., Olivia Wu, Ph.D., and Lilian S. Murray, Ph.D., University of Glasgow — all in Glasgow, Scotland; and Sara Twaddle, Ph.D., Scottish Intercollegiate Guidelines Network, and Gordon D. Murray, Ph.D., University of Edinburgh Medical School. Uterine-Artery embolization versus surgery for symptomatic uterine fibroids. N Engl J Med. 2007;356:360–70.
3. Smeets AJ, Nijenhuis RJ, van Rooij WJ, Weimar EAM, Boekkooi PF, Lampmann LEH, Vervest HAM, Lohle PNM. Uterine artery embolization in patients with a large fibroid burden: long-term clinical and MR follow-up. Cardiovasc Intervent Radiol. 2010;33:943–8.
4. Gupta JK, Sinha AS, Lumsden MA, Hickey M. Uterine artery embolization for symptomatic uterine fibroids. Cochrane Database Syst Rev. 2006;25;(1):CD005073.
5. Li Q, Yang Z-Q, Mohammed W, Feng Y-L, Shi H-B, Zhou X. Prophylactic uterine artery embolization assisted cesarean section for the prevention of intrapartum hemorrhage in high-risk patients. Cardiovasc Intervent Radiol. 2014;37(6):1458–63.
6. Patel SJ, Reede DL, Katz DS, Subramaniam R, Amorosa JK. Imaging the pregnant patient for nonobstetric conditions: algorithms and radiation dose considerations. Radiographics. 2007;27(6):1705–22.
7. Thabet A, Kalva SP, Liu B, Mueller PR, Lee SI. Interventional radiology in pregnancy complications: indications, technique, and methods for minimizing radiation exposure. Radiographics. 2012;32(1):255–74.
8. El-Khoury GY, Madsen MT, Blake ME, Yankowitz J. A new pregnancy policy for a new era. AJR Am J Roentgenol. 2003;181(2):335–40.
9. Schirf BE, Vogelzang RL, Chrisman HB. Complications of uterine fibroid embolization. Semin Intervent Radiol. 2006;23:143–9.

Chapter 7
Miscellaneous Indications for Embolization: Indications for Bleeding or for Decreasing Vascularity in Different Vascular Beds

Abstract In this chapter, we discuss the various indications for vascular embolizations in different vascular beds. Some of these indications range from common conditions like epistaxis to rare conditions like myositis ossificans of the long bones. Embolization of arteriovenous malformations in the head and neck present a technical challenge. Intra-abdominal bleeding due to pseudoaneurysms secondary to pancreatitis are also amenable for embolization. The indications, technical details, complications and outcomes of embolization for epistaxis, arteriovenous malformations and tumours are discussed here.

Keywords Epistaxis • Myositis ossificans • Arterio-venous malformation • Pseudoaneurysm • Bleeding • Pancreatitis

Epistaxis

Most cases of epistaxis are from an anterior source and can be treated with pressure, anterior nasal packing, or cautery. Intractable epistaxis is generally posterior in origin and the site is inaccessible requiring endoscopic cautery, posterior packing, surgical ligation, or embolization. Embolization has been used to treat epistaxis for more than 30 years and success rates have been reported in approximately 90 % of patients, with major complications occurring in approximately 2 %. These excellent results require thorough knowledge of the regional anatomy, familiarity with the equipment and various agents used to achieve this type of embolization, as well as attention to detail and meticulous technique. Several aspects of embolization need attention including the agent of choice, preferred size of the embolic material used, and the number of vessels to be embolized.

Historical Perspective

Epistaxis is a Greek word meaning nosebleed and these records describe the use of the ashes of papyrus mixed with vinegar to treat nasal bleeds. Hippocrates said that pinching the nose "for some time" and asking the patient to breathe through the mouth stopped bleeding from the nose. In 1869, Pilz was the first person to treat

© Springer International Publishing Switzerland 2017

K. Varghese, S. Adhyapak, *Therapeutic Embolization*,
DOI 10.1007/978-3-319-42494-1_7

epistaxis by surgically ligating the external carotid artery. Although in 1879 James Little and Carl Michel were the first to identify the vascular plexus in the anterior part of the nasal septum ("Little's area") as the common area from which nasal bleeding occurs, Wilhelm Kiesselbach's 1884 paper describing the area has led to the common usage of "Kiesselbach plexus" to describe this common source of epistaxis. Seiffert described ligation of the internal maxillary artery (IMAX) through the maxillary antrum via the Caldwell-Luc approach to control epistaxis in 1929 [1].

Sokoloff et al. [2] in 1974 described the successful transcatheter embolization of epistaxis in two patients using Gelfoam (GF) (Gelfoam-Pharmacia and Upjohn Company, Kalamazoo, MI).

Since that time a variety of embolic agents have been used including GF, autologous clot, fat, marrow, polyvinyl alcohol (PVA), calibrated microspheres, N-butyl cyanoacrylate, coils, Onyx, and other agents. The proximity to the brain and eyes makes the endovascular treatment of epistaxis somewhat more challenging and risky than embolization in other locations of the body.

Etiology and Prevalence

Epistaxis is extremely common, occurring in up to 60 % of the adult population at some time in their lives. Approximately 80 % of cases will be caused by an anterior bleeding source [3] with a minority of cases resulting from a posterior source.

Most epistaxis resulting from an anterior source is self-limited with only 6 % requiring medical attention [4]. There is a nearly equal distribution between men and women; however, posterior intractable epistaxis is more common in elderly males. Most large studies show a mild peak in epistaxis cases in the first to second decade of life, and a subsequent increase with age above 40 years. Associated risk factors include hypertension, inflammation/infection (allergic, bacterial, fungal, and viral), medications (e.g., aspirin, nonsteroidal anti-inflammatory drugs, warfarin, and clopidogrel), coagulopathy (e.g., hereditary hemorrhagic telangiectasia [HHT]), postsurgical/iatrogenic injuries, and trauma.

Rarely, other unusual causes such as tumor (e.g., juvenile angiofibroma), aneurysm, or vascular malformation may be causative.

Epistaxis is more common in the winter months. This seasonal variation is believed to be related to reduced humidity, temperature, and increased prevalence of upper respiratory tract infections.

Vascular Anatomy

The blood supply of the nasal cavity is rich and varied. The nasal fossa is supplied by both the internal carotid artery (ICA) and the external carotid artery (ECA) (Fig. 7.1). The dominant supply in most individuals is from the ECA via distal branches of the internal maxillary artery (IMAX). Several authors also describe a small contribution

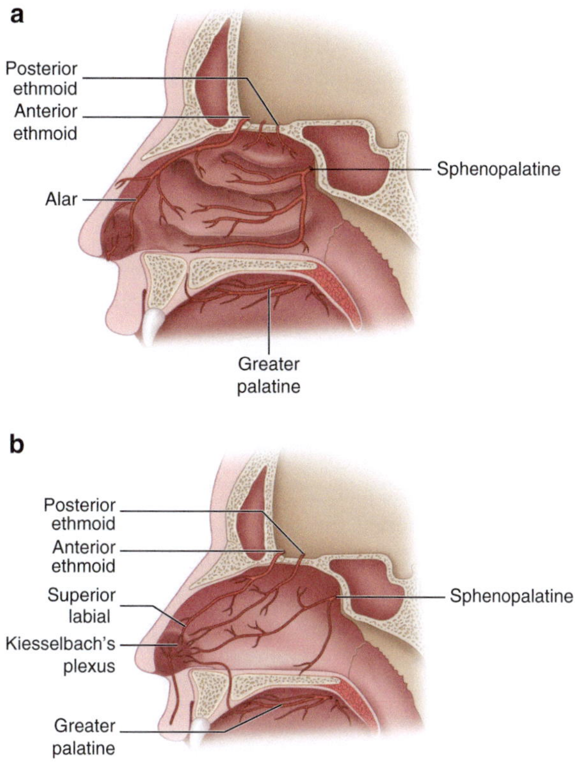

Fig. 7.1 Schematic arterial anatomy of the nasal cavity. (**a**) Medial nasal wall shows blood supply of nasal septum. (**b**) Blood supply of lateral nasal wall. Kiesselbach plexus (or Little area), the site of most anterior epistaxis, is noted

to the posterior nasal cavity from the ascending pharyngeal artery (APhA), which arises from the IMAX just beyond the facial artery (FA) origin. Important branches of the IMAX include the sphenopalatine artery (SPA) and the greater palatine artery (GPA). The GPA is the terminal branch of the descending palatine artery (DPA). The SPA provides the dominant supply to the nasal cavity walls via both medial (septal) and lateral branch; the lateral branch supplies the superior, middle, and inferior turbinates, while the medial branch supplies the nasal septum. The richly vascularized posterior aspect of the nasal cavity, sometimes referred to as Woodruff plexus, is primarily supplied by the SPA. The GPA courses via the incisive foramen to supply the inferior portion (floor) of the nasal septum and anastomoses with septal branches of the SPA. The FA generally supplies the more anteroinferior portion of the nasal cavity via the terminal alar branches of the superior labial artery (SLA) as well as the lateral nasal artery (LNA). ICA supply to the nasal cavity is most often by the ophthalmic artery (OphA) via the anterior ethmoidal artery (AEA) and posterior ethmoidal artery (PEA). The ethmoidal arteries course through the cribriform plate to supply the roof of the nasal cavity and communicate with branches of the SPA posteriorly and several other arteries anteriorly. Due to their diminutive size, the ethmoidal arteries are rarely seen on normal arteriograms. Kiesselbach plexus is a highly vascularized region at the anteroinferior nasal septum. It is the sight of most anterior epistaxis and is richly supplied via braches of the AEA, PEA, SPA, GPA, and SLA/alar branches of the FA.

As the IMAX is the critical vessel in most cases of epistaxis, it is absolutely necessary the angiographer to have a complete knowledge of the anatomy of the IMAX. The IMAX is the larger of the two terminal branches of the external carotid artery, with the other being the superficial temporal artery (STA). The IMAX arises behind the neck of the mandible, travels through the substance of the parotid gland, and passes forward between the ramus of the mandible and the sphenomandibular ligament. It courses either superficial or deep to the lateral pterygoid muscle to the pterygopalatine fossa.

The IMAX is classically divided into three segments termed the mandibular, pterygoid, and pterygopalatine segments. The branches of segment 1 (mandibular) include the deep auricular, anterior tympanic, inferior alveolar, middle meningeal (MMA), and accessory meningeal (AccMA) arteries. These proximal branches of the IMAX may be recalled using the mnemonic "MIADA." It is critical to identify the proximal segmental branches, as they are a common pathway for ECA–ICA collateralization, especially in cases of ICA obstruction/stenosis. The second or pterygoid portion of the IMAX courses obliquely forward and upward under the mandibular ramus and insertion of the temporalis on the surface of the lateral pterygoid muscle; it then passes between the two heads of origin of this muscle and enters the pterygoid fossa. Branches include the masseteric artery, pterygoid branches, posterior deep temporal artery, and buccal artery. This large contribution to the muscles of mastication in conjunction with proximity to branches supplying the nasal cavity explains the common incidence of jaw claudication following IMAX embolization. The anterior deep temporal artery may arise from the distal second or proximal third portion of the IMAX.

The third or pterygopalatine portion of the IMAX contains the important contributors to epistaxis as well as other branches. These include the DPA (which branches into the GPA and lesser palatine artery), posterior superior alveolar artery, pharyngeal artery, artery of the pterygoid canal (vidian artery), infraorbital artery (IOA) (most anterior branch of IMAX), middle and superior alveolar arteries (both branches of the IOA), and the SPA, which is generally the terminal branch of the IMAX.

In cases of epistaxis, it is also important to consider the FA anatomy. The FA generally arises from the ventral surface of the ECA and courses inside the mandible.

Near its origin, the FA gives rise to the ascending palatine artery (APA). The FA turns downward and forward as it passes around the mandible and gives off tonsillar and small glandular branches (i.e., submandibular artery), and the submental artery. The FA becomes superficial and subcutaneous, courses cephalad along the mandible in a variable direction, and gives rise to the inferior labial artery. The FA ascends to the maxilla and gives rise to the SLA; the SLA supplies the anterior nasal septum and gives rise to alar branches to the nasal ala. The FA courses superiorly and slightly posterior and gives rise to the LNA, supplying the ala and lateral nose. The FA gives rise to the angular artery (AngA) in its terminal segment.

The AngA anastomoses with the dorsal nasal branch (DNA) of the OphA. Along its course, the FA also variably supplies muscular branches to the internal pterygoid, stylohyoid, masseter, and buccinator.

Important Anastomoses

It is critical to understand the anastomoses between the ECA and the ICA when performing arteriography and/or embolization in this region. The ECA, ICA, and OphA have important anastomoses that are always present but often not visualized or recognized on standard arteriography. Well-described anastomoses between the ECA and ICA include the vidian artery, inferolateral trunk ((ILT)—supplies the artery of foramen rotundum and the artery of foramen ovale), and meningohypophyseal trunk. Other important ECA–ICA collateral pathways, especially when the ICA is obstructed, include MMA, AccMA, and APhA. ECA collateralization to the OphA or to the ICA retrograde via the OphA is also important to assess. In a small number of individuals, the ECA may provide the dominant supply to the OphA. Well-known but often poorly visualized collateral pathways exist between the SPA, FA, and OphA. The IOA is particularly noteworthy in this regard, as it may anastomoses with the terminal branches of the FA (LNA, SLA, and AngA), DNA branch of OphA, transverse facial artery ((TFA)-most proximal branch of the STA), and buccal arteries.

The FA also has a rich network of anastomoses. Important anastomoses exist between the APA and the DPA, APhA, and AccMA. Several FA branches, including the LNA and AngA, may anastomose with the TFA. The SLA and LNA anastomose with each other. The LNA anastomoses with the septal and alar branches of the SLA, with the DNA of the OphA, and with the IOA branch of the IMAX. The AngA anastomoses with the DNA.

These collateral pathways make it imperative that the interventionalist performs high-quality, high-resolution arteriography to exclude visible anastomoses as these communications are not seen on initial arteriography often. It must be kept in mind that during embolization, as flow is altered, collateral pathways may open up and be a source of emboli to the ICA or OphA. Therefore, a thorough knowledge of the vascular anatomy, high resolution angiography and vigilance is required during the procedure.

Embolization Technique and Results

Successful control of intractable epistaxis hinges on control of the bleeding source. The arteriogram will generally not reveal an active site of bleeding. Common carotid arteriography (CCA), generally performed via a 5 F catheter or 5/6 F guiding catheter, may be useful to evaluate the carotid bulb and bifurcation area prior to selective catheterizations. Most practitioners strongly advocate performance of high-resolution digital subtraction angiography of both the ICA and ECA [2, 5]. While active bleeding is only rarely evident on the arteriogram in idiopathic epistaxis, hyperemia, blush, or increased vascularity may be appreciated [6–9]. Arteriograms in cases of trauma or tumor will more commonly reveal abnormal findings such as pseudoaneurysm, active bleeding, or puddling of contrast. Rarely, an arteriovenous malformation (AVM) or arteriovenous fistula (AVF) may be detected. The ICA arteriogram 38 will serve to exclude dangerous collaterals and exclude rare ICA sources of bleeding as described above (e.g., carotid cavernous fistula [CCF], cavernous carotid artery aneurysm [CCAA], [10, 11] and AVM) [12]. A careful search should be undertaken to identify the dominant supply to the OphA and for contributions to the nasal cavity. from the AEA or PEA. The ECA arteriogram will detail the anatomy of the important supply to the nasal cavity (SPA, GPA, FA, AEA, etc.) as well as the many other potential collaterals to both the nasal cavity and the ICA. If the ECA is the dominant supply to the OphA, embolization is relatively contraindicated due to the risk of blindness.

Once the ICA and ECA have been completely evaluated, most operators will place a microcatheter (0.018–0.028 ID) into the IMAX. The microcatheter may be placed via the 5 F diagnostic catheter or via a 5 of 6 F guide catheter. Detailed IMAX arteriography may be performed via the microcatheter. The microcatheter is advanced as distally as possible into the pterygopalatine segment of the IMAX beyond the AccMA and MMA. Most of the literature describes embolization with use of PVA or GF.

Both agents have a long track record for safety and efficacy throughout the vascular system and in the treatment of epistaxis [3, 13]. Multiple reports describe their favorable safety profile [12, 14–16]. Most reports describe use of PVA particles in the 150–350 μm range and GF in the 1–3 mm range. Although the use of smaller particles (50–150 μm) is described, this may lead to increased risk of ischemia [7, 17] or have a higher risk of non-target embolization via collateral vessels. Thirty five Slightly larger size particles may be useful when treating FAs to prevent skin necrosis [17]. The distal IMAX embolization is performed until there is near stagnation of antegrade flowand nomore visualization of the nasal blush. Coil embolization is generally not done for epistaxis except to prevent non-target embolization and when use of particulate material is not possible. In cases of FA embolization, larger particles are used to prevent non-target embolization and prevent ischemia. The use of gelfoam has been advocated in this situation (Figs. 7.2 and 7.3).

Results of Embolization

The results of embolization have reported 86–90 % success [3, 7, 16].

Minor complications related to epistaxis embolization are generally mild, self-limited, and related primarily to ischemia of the nasal region. These include temporofacial pain or numbness, headache, swelling, jaw claudication, and less commonly trismus.

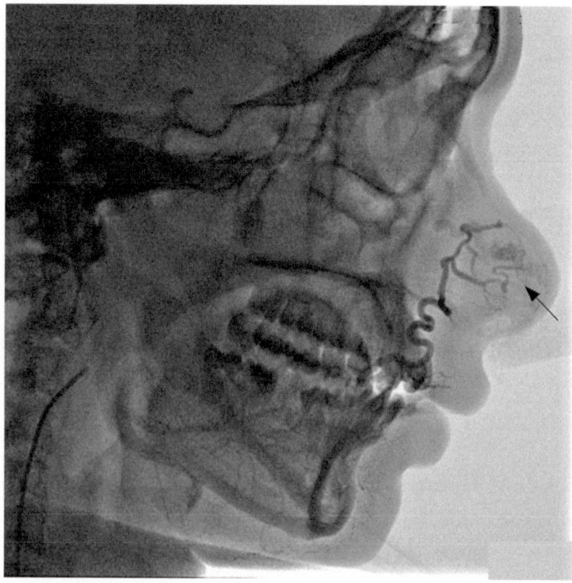

Fig. 7.2 Selective cannulation of the facial artery demonstrating an AV malformation of the nose (*arrow*)

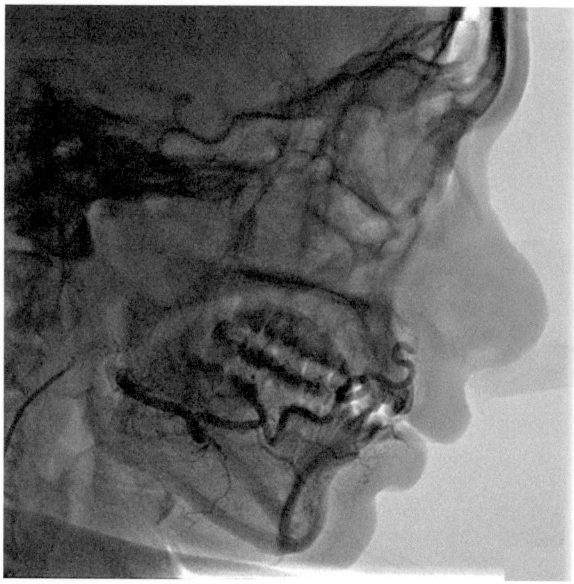

Fig. 7.3 Obliteration of the arterio-venous malformation by selective injection of PVA particles. The post-embolization angiogram demonstrates sluggish flow in the feeding artery to the arterio- venous malformation with disappearance of the arterio-venous malformation

Major complications include skin necrosis [7, 17] facial nerve paralysis, [18] monocular blindness, and cerebrovascular accident [12].

The variability in reporting and technique make it difficult to draw conclusions regarding optimal technique. But, the rate of complications increases linearly with the number of vessels embolized. The rate of complications is therefore greater in patients who undergo bilateral embolization for bleeding.

Tumors of the Nasopharynx

Epistaxis may be seen in a variety of neoplasms that involve the nasosinus. These include, but are not limited to, juvenile nasopharyngeal angiofibroma (JNA) [19] (Figs. 7.4 and 7.5); nasopharyngeal carcinoma [20, 21]; adenoid cystic neoplasm; acute myelogenous leukemia; malignant fibrous histiocytoma; pyogenic granuloma; hemangioma; hemangiopericytoma; meningioma [22]; and metastases. JNA, most often seen in males in the second decade of life, represent highly vascular tumors with a propensity for local spread via the skull base. JNA is one of the more common tumors that may present with epistaxis; definitive treatment of JNA relies primarily on complete surgical removal [23, 24]. Embolization for JNA has been described to treat acute epistaxis [25] and in the preoperative setting to reduce tumour vascularity [24]. Technique is similar to that described for idiopathic epistaxis, with the exception that when deemed safe, smaller particles (50–150 μm) may be used to affect greater devascularization of the tumor [26].

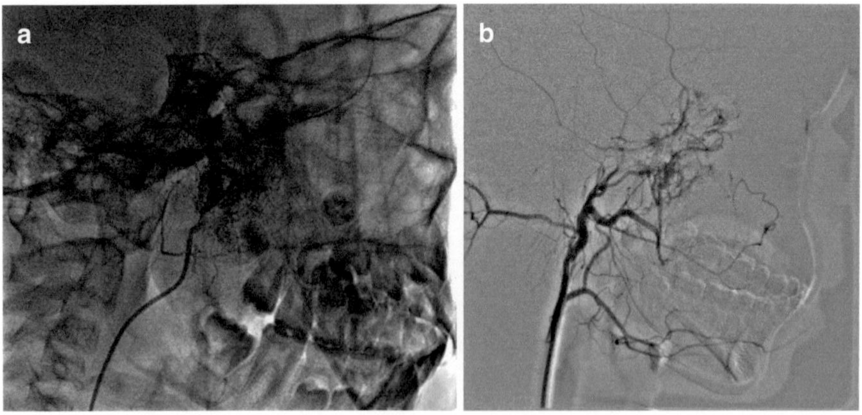

Fig. 7.4 (**a**) Selective cannulation of the external maxillary artery demonstrates a vascular tumor/mass in the nose. (**b**) Digital subtraction angiography demonstrating the same

Maxillofacial Trauma

Maxillofacial trauma is usually treated surgically. Some patients treated initially with surgery may still require embolization in case of failure of ligation [27]. Angiography is used to identify the exact source of bleeding [28] and to help facilitate embolization. Trauma patients may also present in a delayed fashion secondary to pseudoaneurysm formation and less commonly due to arteriovenous fistula formation. Particulate embolic agents may be used in many cases, but microcoils have more often been described in the setting of vessel laceration or pseudoaneurysm formation (Figs. 7.6, 7.7, 7.8, and 7.9).

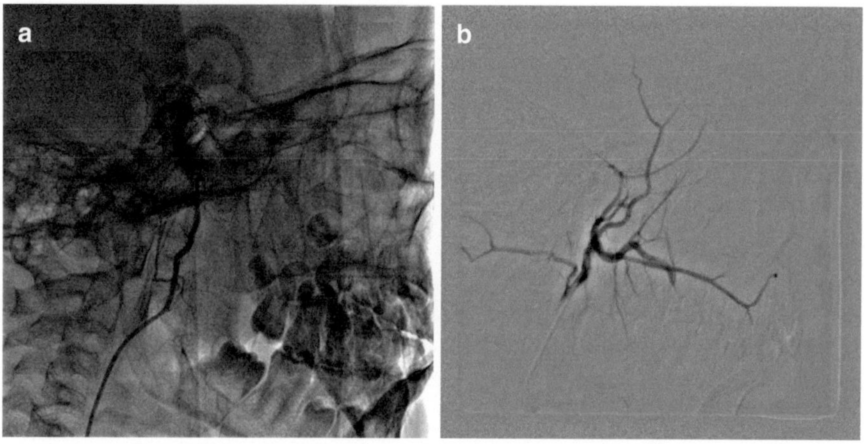

Fig. 7.5 (**a**) Post-embolization angiogram demonstrates decrease in vascularity of the nasal tumor. (**b**) Digital subtraction angiography demonstrating the same

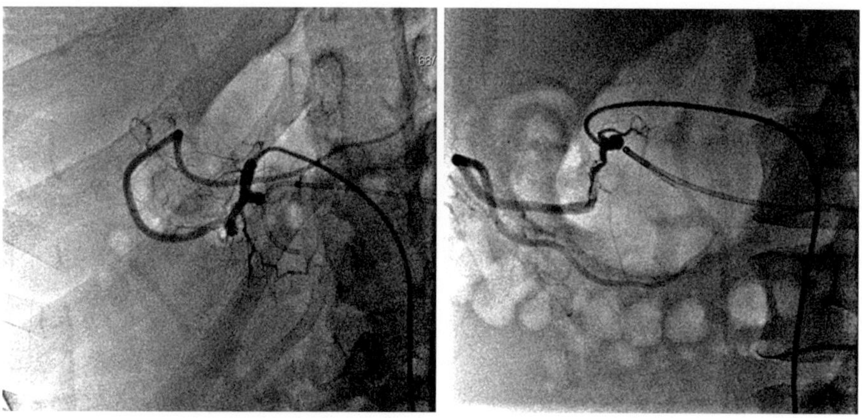

Figs. 7.6 and 7.7 Angiography performed using a catheter introduced via the coeliac artery into the gastroduodenal arterydemonstrating a discrete aneurysm in the gastro-duodenal artery. The catheter has been advanced till the aneurysm

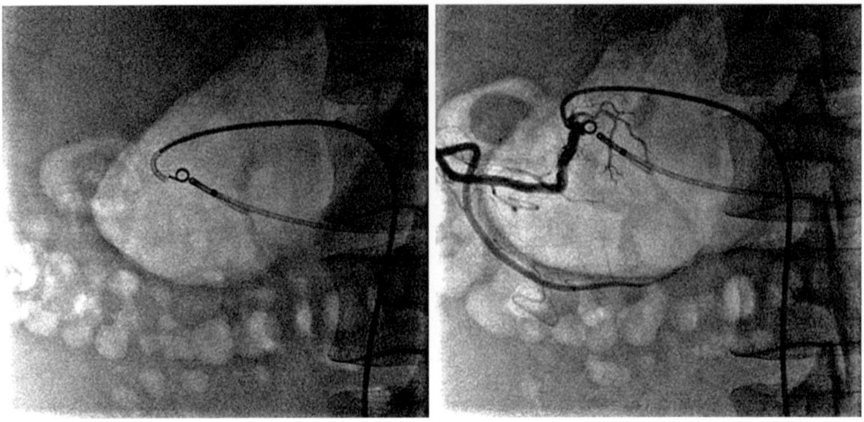

Figs. 7.8 and 7.9 A coil has been deployed into the aneurysm with successful thrombosis and occlusion of the aneurysm

Our Experience

We have performed transcatheter embolization for posterior epistaxis and for devascularizing nasopharyngeal angiofibromas prior to surgical excision. We have had a 98 % success rate with 0 % complications and a recurrence rate of 0.1 %.

Trancatheter embolization is effective in certain cases of posterior epistaxis with an 86–90 % success rate and has associated complications. Operator expertise, proper imaging and use of proper embolization materials are essential for procedural success and for minimizing complication rates. It is also effective in devascularizing tumors of the nasopharynx prior to surgical excision. Rarely, it can be used for specific indications in maxillofacial trauma.

Myositis Ossificans

Introduction

Myositis ossificans is a well known benign ossifying process occurring most commonly in the muscle or sometimes in other soft parts [29]. The pathogenesis of myositis ossificans is not well understood [30]. This phenomenon of unknown etiology occurs after damage to muscles with subsequent proliferation of connective tissue and differentiation into mature bone [31].

Etiology and Pathogenesis

It is assumed that tissue necrosis leads to heterotrophic fibroblastic and vascular proliferation with eventual ossification [30]. Trauma has been associated with the majority of cases, although there are reported cases without an antecedent injury [30]. The most reported risk-factor is re-injury during the early stages of recovery [31]. Causes that have been cited are acute sports injuries, such as in American football, and repetitive occupational trauma, such as in the cavalrymen and shoemakers [32].

Clinical Features

It usually affects young males. Symptoms are of pain and deformity of the involved limb. Clinically, they may be seen as an outgrowth from the shaft of the femur or tibia. The X-rays show an outer layer of dense bone covering a cancellous structure. As this is ectopic ossification of soft tissue, these are amenable to surgical removal. As they contain osteblasts, fibroblasts and vascular tissue, they tend to be vascular.

Indications for Embolization

As these lesions are vascular, pre-operative devascularization is indicated in large lesions. As they usually involve long shaft bones of the limbs, selective catheterization and angiography reveals a vascular blush with abnormal collaterals. The embolization materials used are usually gelfoam or slightly larger PVA particles (250–400 μm). Post-embolization angiograms should document disappearance of the vascular blush and collaterals. Subtotal embolization should be the goal, as complete embolization can lead to non-target embolization and limb ischemia.

Complications

The complication rates are related to procedural technique with non-target embolization due to reflux of embolization material and complete embolization of the involved vasculature.

Our Experience

We have performed pre-operative embolization for myositis ossificans with a 97 % success rate, 0 % complication and 0 % recurrence rate (Figs. 7.10, 7.11, 7.12, and 7.13).

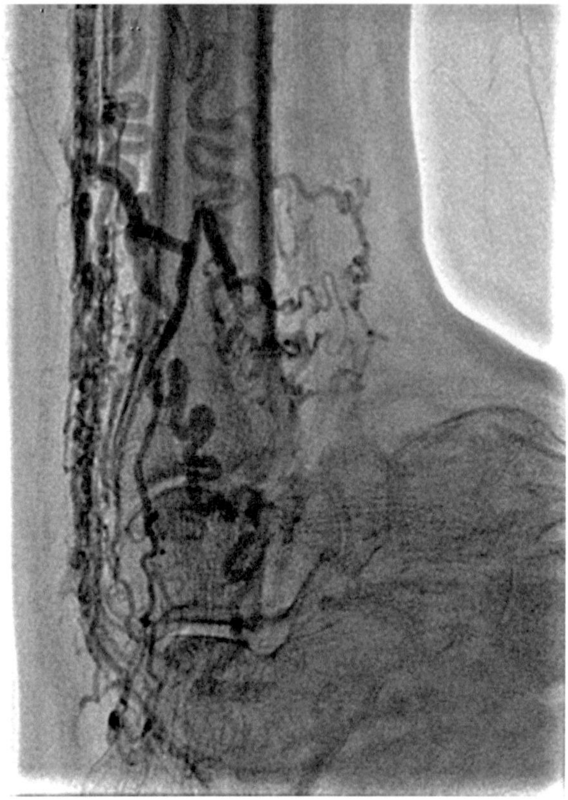

Fig. 7.10 Selective injection into the posterior tibial artery demonstrating an AVM the foot

Arteriovenous Malformations

Definition

Arteriovenous malformations (AVMs) are congenital highflow vascular malformations composed of anomalous capillary beds shunting blood from the arterial system to the venous system.

Natural Course

Puberty and trauma trigger the growth of congenital AVMs and enhance the manifestation of its troublesome symptoms [33]. They are infiltrative causing destruction of local tissue and often life-threatening secondary to massive bleeding. Some AVMs occur following trauma in adults and are secondary to certain disease processes like pancreatitis.

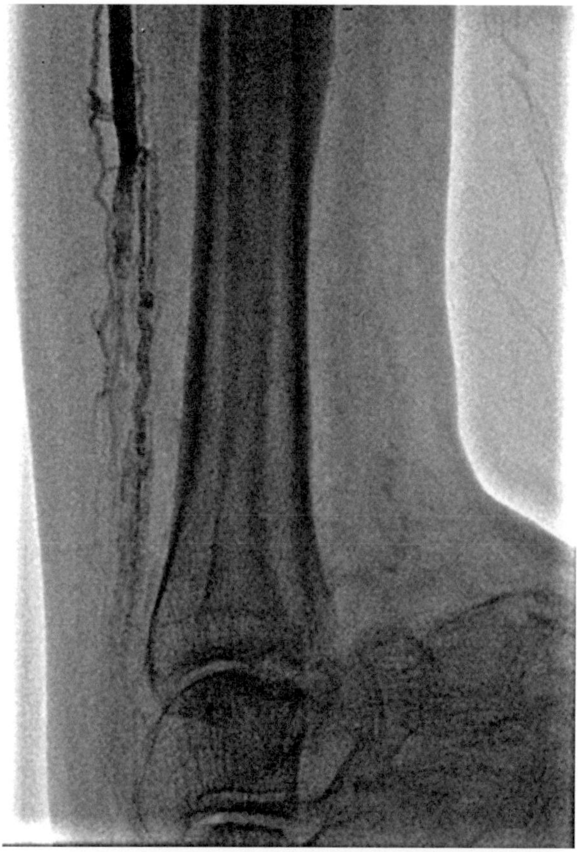

Fig. 7.11 Post-embolization angiogram demonstrating sluggish flow and disappearance of the abnormal vasculature

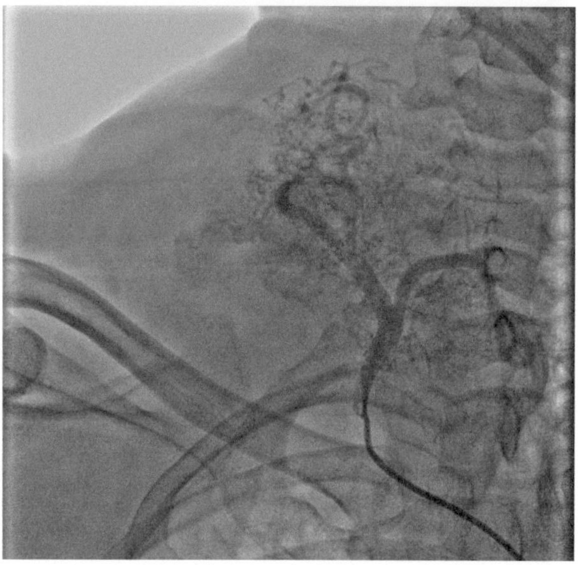

Fig. 7.12 Selective injection of a vascular mass in the neck (tumor) showing vascular blush

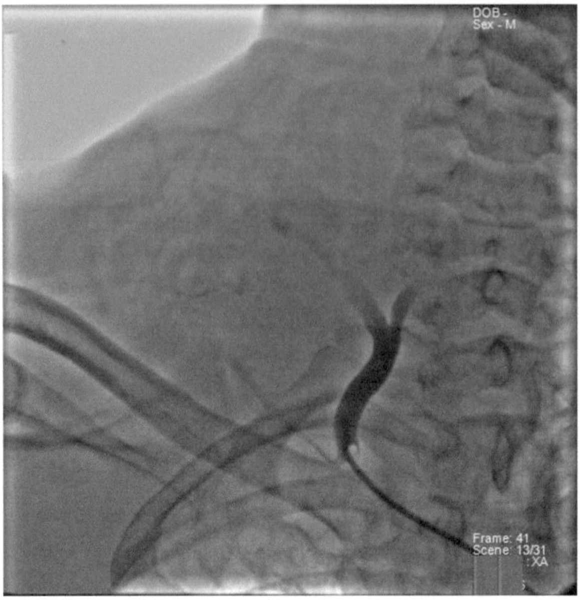

Fig. 7.13 Post-embolization angiogram demonstrating occlusion of the feeder vessel

The natural course of congenital AVM is early quiescence, late expansion, and ultimately infiltration and destruction of local soft tissue and bone. Common sites for occurrence are the midface, oral cavity, and limbs [33]. AVMs are by far the most difficult vascular anomaly to manage due to the replacement of normal tissue by disease vessels and very high recurrence rates [34, 35].

Diagnosis

Imaging is essential in identifying the extent of AVM. MRI may be useful, but MRA and CTA can give a superior outline of these lesions [36]. Numerous hypolucent arterial flow voids are the hallmark of AVM by MRI. CTA allows evaluation of surrounding tissues and bones. Individual arterial feeders can be visualized with this imaging as well [37]. An arteriogram, the time-tested approach to diagnosing AVM, will provide good definition of central "nidus" of affected vessels and provide access for intravascular treatment when necessary [38].

Treatment

Treatment of AVM consists of embolization, surgical extirpation, or a combination of these modalities. Treatment and timing are often individualized to the patient and the extent of disease. For example, small-vessel AVMs are known to be localized and can be resected with good long-term outcomes [39]. Intravascular embolization of AVM can be used alone or in combination with surgical excision. Absolute ethanol, polyvinyl alcohol, and ONYX have been employed as AVM embolization materials [40]. These agents selectively obstruct and destroy the arteries treated (Figs. 7.14, 7.15, 7.16, 7.17, 7.18, 7.19, 7.20, 7.21, 7.22, 7.23, 7.24, and 7.25). Complications are due to non-target embolization and include tissue necrosis. Therefore, the use of ethanol and ONYX has been abandoned for AVM embolization. The use of PVA particles and gelfoam is recommended. Embolization provides temporary control of disease, but recurrence is high [41]. This is theoretically due to collateralization and recruitment of new vessels to support an undetected portion of the "nidus." Frequent serial embolizations may improve patient outcomes.

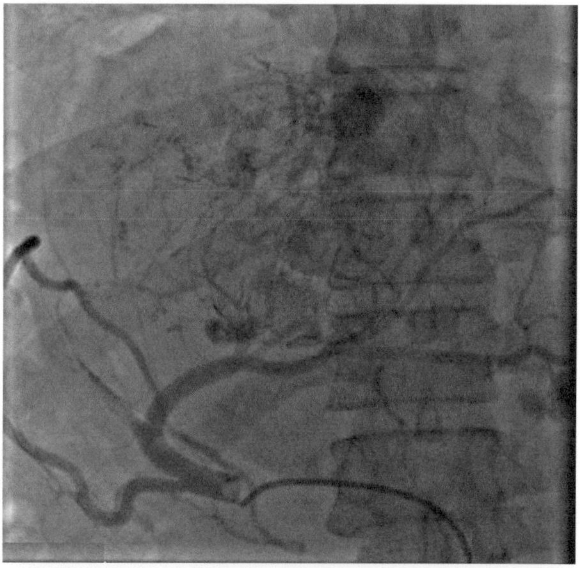

Fig. 7.14 Angiogram of the hepatic artery in a patient with hepatocellular carcinoma demonstrating areas of tumor blush

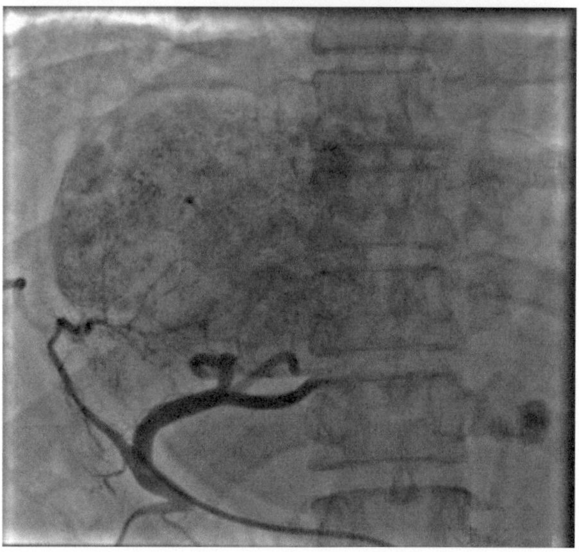

Fig. 7.15 PostembolizationAngiogram. Chemoembolization was done using Lipiodol mixed with a chemotherapeutic agent followed by Gelfoam embolization

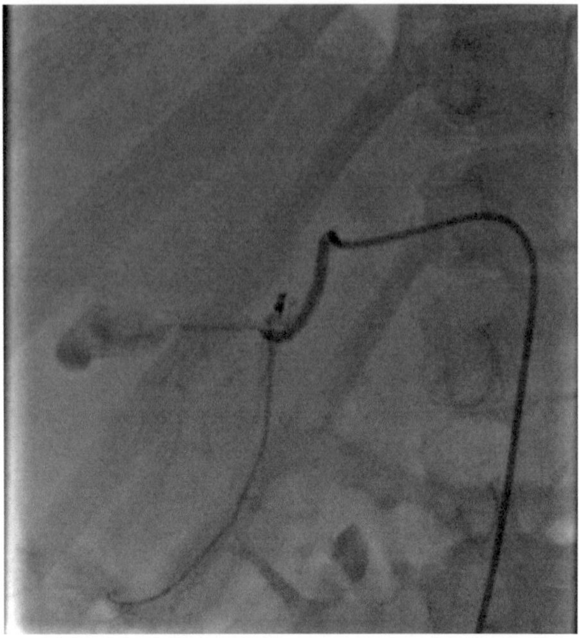

Fig. 7.16 Selective angiogram of the hepatic artery in a patient with hemobilia demonstrating a large seudoaneurysm

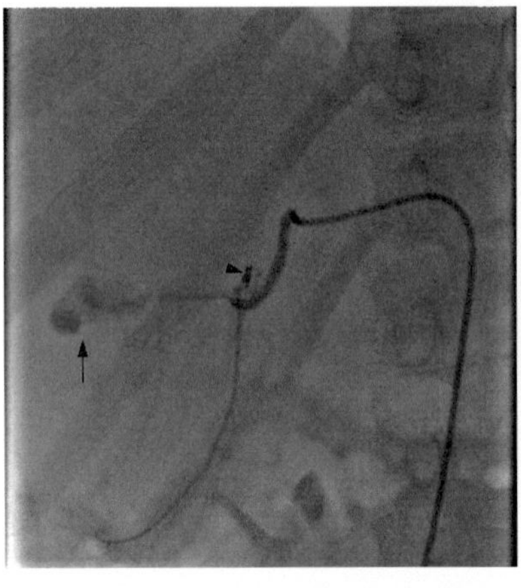

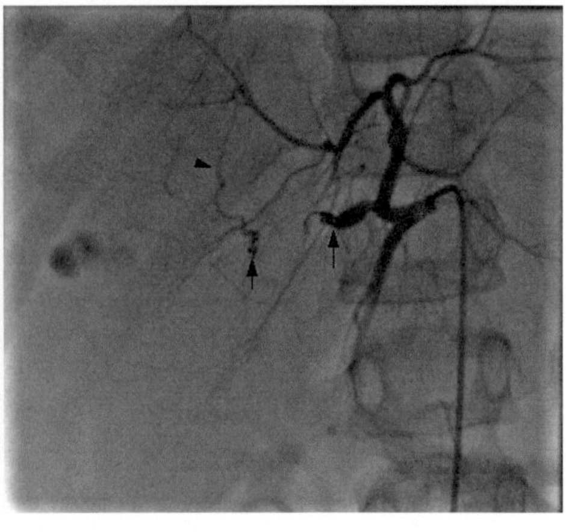

Figs. 7.17 and 7.18 Post-embolization angiograms. Obliteration of the Pseudoaneurysm (*vertical arrow*) was achieved by first deploying a smaller coil (*arrowhead*) distal to the origin of the feeding artery. Fig 7.18 shows the locations of the two coils (*vertical arrows*). If only proximal occlusion was performed, the pseudoaneurysm would have persisted due to collateral blood supply (*arrowhead*) thus demonstrating the need to occlude proximal and distal to the origin of the feeding artery

In general, surgical management of AVMs requires preoperative supraselective embolization, judicious removal of tissue, and complex reconstructive techniques. In focal lesions, surgical excision has been shown to cure AVM [35, 42]. However, diffuse AVMs have recurrence rates as high as 93 %[41]. Excision is preformed 24–48 h after embolization. This helps control blood loss and delineate the surgical margins of the lesion.

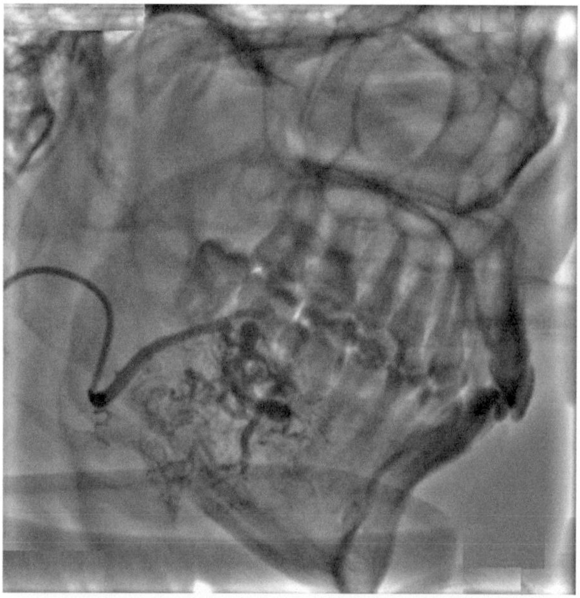

Fig. 7.19 Angiogram of the mandibular artery demonstrating a large AVM

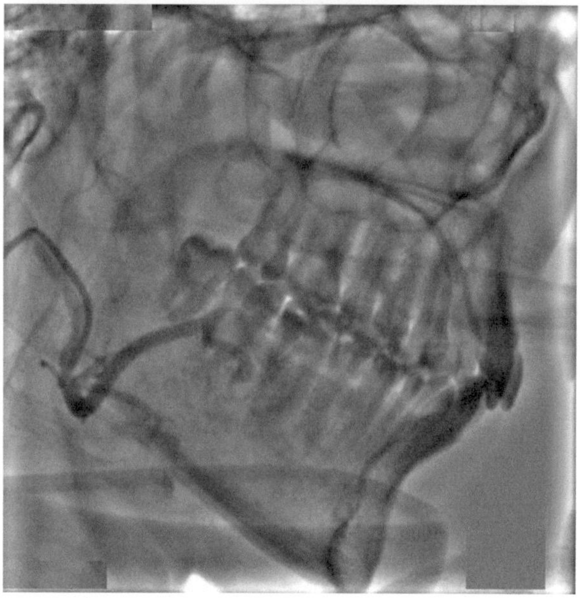

Fig. 7.20 Post-embolization angiogram showing absence of the AVM

Pulmonary AVM

Pulmonary arteriovenous malformations (PAVMs) are fistulous shunts of high-grade flow between the pulmonary artery and vein. More than 80 % of the cases are congenital, but they may appear secondary to acquired conditions such as liver cirrhosis, schistosomiasis, mitral stenosis, trauma, actinomycosis, metastatic thyroid carcinoma, and bronchiectasis [43].

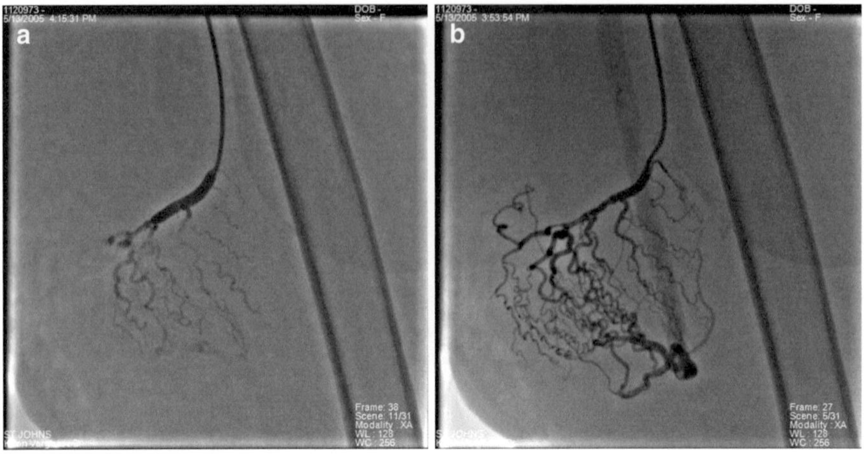

Fig. 7.21 Preoperative embolizationof a patient with myositis ossificans in the thigh. Angiography before (**a**) and after (**b**) gelfoam embolization showing marked reduction in vascularity

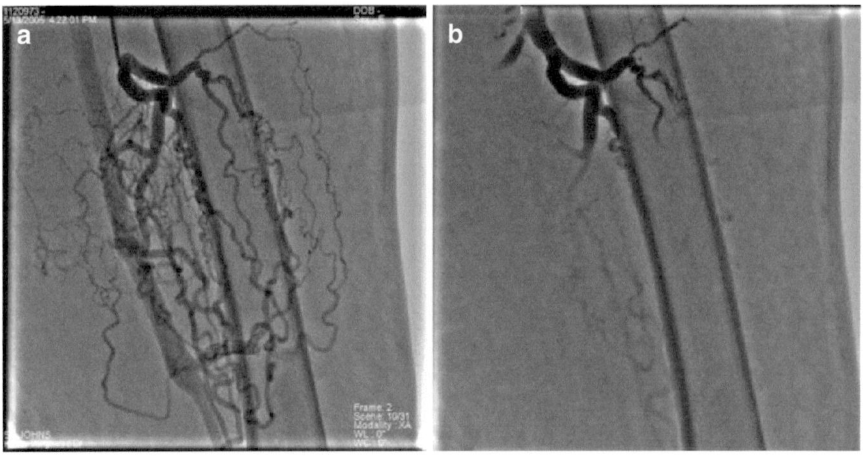

Fig. 7.22 Markedly increased vascularity (**a**) with reduction in vascularity following embolization (**b**)

PAVM is divided into two types : simple and complicated types [44]. In the simple type, a single feeding artery connects to a drainage vein, whereas in the complicated type, there are two or more feeding vessels and/or drainage veins. Surgery and embolotherapy are two approaches in the management of PAVM [45].

Management

As upto 40 % of PAVMs are diagnosed during the diagnostic work-up for neurological disorders like migraine attacks (43 %), transient ischemic attacks (37 %), stroke (18 %), brain abscesses (9 %) and epileptic seizures (8 %) [46–48]. Therefore,

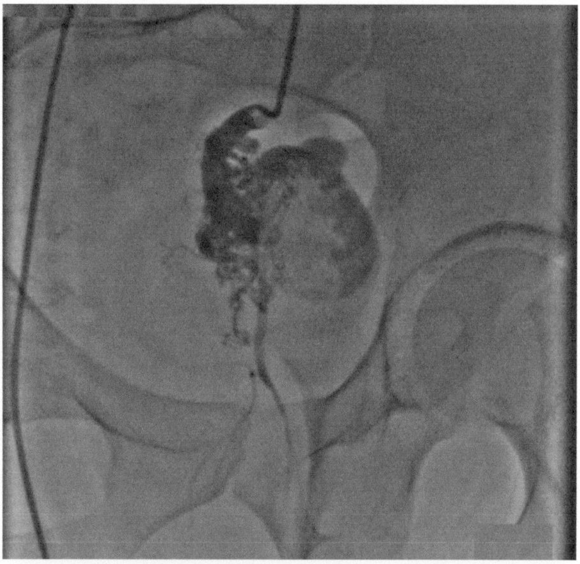

Fig. 7.23 Selective angiogram of the contralateral internal iliac artery demonstrating a large AVM

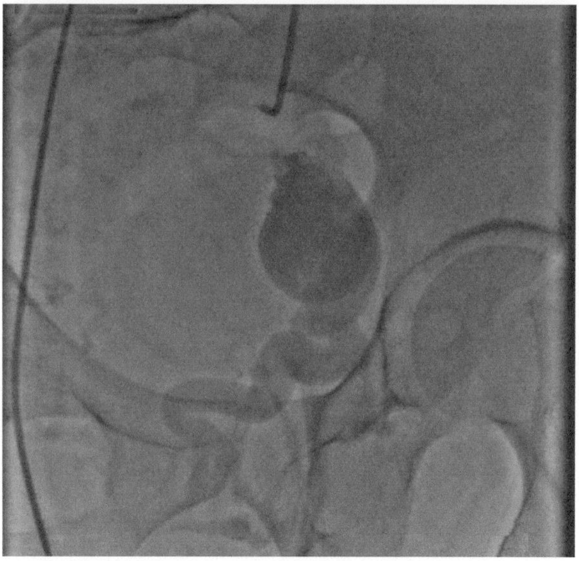

Fig. 7.24 Selective angiogram of the contralateral internal iliac artery demonstrating the venous phase of a large AVM

treatment of every case with PAVM, whether symptomatic or asymptomatic, is the recommended management approach [49, 50].

Until Talor et al. reported the first successful percutaneous embolization in 1978 [51], surgical techniques like local excision, segmental resection, lobectomy, ligation, and pneumectomy were used for the treatment of PAVM [43].

As surgery has its attendant complications, percutaneous embolization is the first treatment of choice for PAVMs. Besides, surgical excision of a complex PAVM needs extensive resection to ligate all the feeder vessels to the AVM.

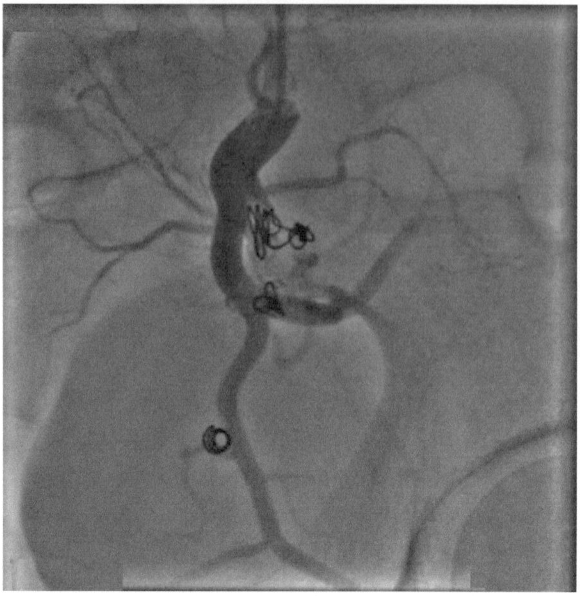

Fig. 7.25 Post-embolization of the AVM with coils (*Arrows*)

Detachable balloons and mechanical coils were used for embolization, however the most extensively used material is the mechanical coil. With regard to radial force, stainless steel has more strength and could be used in fistulas with high-grade of flow, although, due to its strength, it has the risk of perforation and other complications. When PAVMs contain venous sacs, embolization of the sacs with controlled detachable coils like Guglielmi detachable coils may allow safety embolization afterwards [48].

Major Complications

Lung infarct and systemic coil embolization, which are considered major complications, are encountered in 4 % of cases. The dual blood supply of the lungs prevents underlying ischemic infarcts if the embolized area is small. Coil migration, however, is related to technique and incorrect histoanatomical analysis of the PAVM. Contrary to general belief, coil migration and recanalization is encountered more often in simple PAVMs with one feeding artery and one drainage vein [48] than in complicated PAVMs because a thin, permeable capillary membrane structure is absent in simple PAVMs, but present in complicated PAVMs [52].

Minor Complications

Fever, chest pain and pleurisy are seen in around 10–15 % and are self-limiting.

In order to prevent coil migration, coils which are 30 % greater than the diameter of the feeding artery are used for embolization. There are two mechanisms of coil recanalisation.

The first is embolization of a fistula that is too proximal. In this situation, development of a more distal collateral pathway not only causes recanalization, but may prevent further embolization.

This can be overcome by placing the coil as distally as possible in the fistula.

The other cause of recanalization is placement of an insufficient amount of coils. This is overcome by placing several coils in the fistula, especially in the venous sac if present, such that contrast is prevented from seeping between them. This has to be confirmed in two orthogonal projection angiograms.

Our Experience

We have performed coil embolization in five patients with PAVMs. Two patients had simple PAVM and three had complex PAVM. There was a venous sac in all three complex PAVM which was embolized using several coils and a vascular plug in one of them (Figs. 7.26 and 7.27). There were no complications in all five patients with 0 % recurrence rates.

Gastroduodenal AVMs and Pseudoaneurysms

The incidence of visceral vascular aneurysms, pseudoaneurysms and AVMs detected by angiography in chronic pancreatitis is 10 % [53]. Depending on the

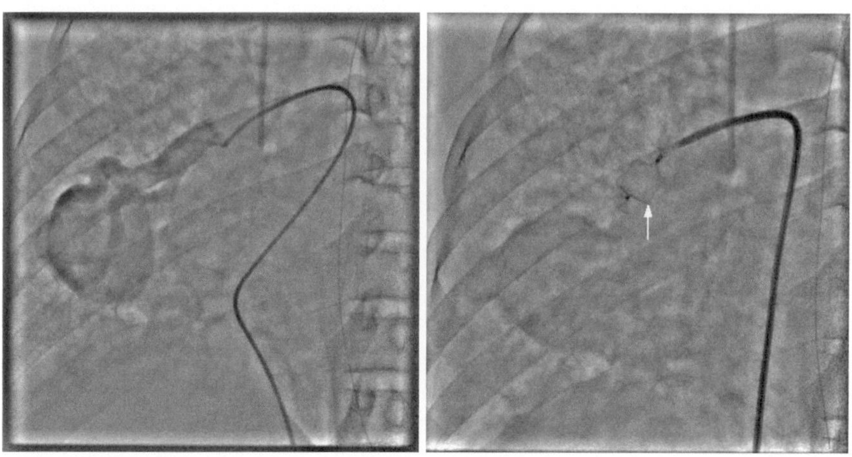

Figs. 7.26 and 7.27 Pulmonary angiogram demonstrating a pulmonary AVM and post-embolizationangiogram showing closure of the AVM with a vascular plug (*arrow*)

mechanism of formation and etiologic factors, they are classified into true aneurysms or pseudoaneurysms.

True aneurysms are the results of vessel wall abnormalities while pseudoaneurysms occur after vascular injuries or erosions such as in trauma or inflammation [53], (i.e., pancreatitis, autoimmune disorders, vascular intervention, laparoscopic cholecystectomy and hepatic transplantation) [54].

Pseudoaneurysms are more common in middle age and are found between 50 and 58 years of age [55, 56]. The male/female ratio is 4.5:1 and the mean size 3.6 cm [55].

They have been reported in almost all the visceral arteries [57] but are most commonly seen in the splenic artery (46 %), followed by the renal artery (22 %), the hepatic artery (16.2 %) and the pancreaticoduodenal artery (1.3 %) [58]. Those involving the gastroduodenal artery comprise only 1.5 % of all reported VAA [53] and most of them are pseudoaneurysms due to their high occurrence rates in the setting of pancreatitis. Pancreatitis was found to be the most common associated condition with gastroduodenal artery aneurysm accounting for 47 % of all cases followed by ethanol abuse (25 %), peptic ulcer disease (17 %) and cholecystectomy (3 %) [53, 57, 59].

The collaterals which develop in celiac artery aneurysms can define the etiology of the aneurysm as congenital or atherosclerotic. The collateral vessels that form early on have usually parallel walls, are of uniform caliber and are limited to one or two vessels. In contrary, arteriosclerotic collaterals are more abundant, dilated and tortuous and hence more prone to aneursymal formation within the vessel's wall. This occurs regardless of the location of the stenosis [60].

The pancreaticoduodenal artery is the main collateral pathway between the celiac axis and the superior mesenteric artery. Increased blood flow in the pancreaticoduodenal artery, as compensation for celiac artery stenosis, may cause a pancreaticoduodenal artery aneurysm [61].

Inflammation with the most common cause being pancreatitis, results in vascular wall destruction that is mediated by pancreatic proteolytic enzymes leading to pseudoaneurysm formation [62].

Clinical Presentation

Gastrointestinal hemorrhage secondary to rupture of the aneurysm was found to be the most common clinical presentation (52 %) while only 7.5 % of GDA aneurysms remained asymptomatic. Abdominal pain is the second most common symptom and occurs in 46 % of cases. The mortality rate with rupture is about 40 % [63] and depends on the severity, speed of the blood loss and the anatomical site of the rupture. The highest mortality rate comes from rupture into the duodenum approaching 21 % [64, 65]. These patients present with hematemesis, melena, and hemodynamic shock [66].

Diagnosis

Imaging studies such as sonography, CT scans and MRI can delineate the vascular pathology. CT scans and MRI have greater specificity. Visceral angiography defines the exact location and nature of the pathology facilitating embolotherapy.

Treatment

Endovascular embolization is an effective alternative therapeutic approach for patients with severe co-morbidities precluding surgical ligation and also offers a shorter hospital stay.

Celiac trunk angiograms and superior mesenteric artery angiograms are done to demonstrate the pseudo aneurysm. A superselective angiography of the gastroduodenal artery may be necessary.

When extravasation of contrast material was demonstrated at angiography, embolic therapy can be performed as selectively as possible, with a microcatheter coaxially inserted through the 5-French catheter into the target vessel.

The embolic agents used are temporary, such as gelfoam and 355- to 500-mm or 500- to 710-mm polyvinyl alcohol particles or permanent, such as vascular coils ranging from 2 to 7 mm

If direct entry into the bleeding artery is not possible, occlusion can be attempted by means of a flow directed injection of the embolic agent. When a dual blood supply exists, contrast injection through the alternate route can be performed to exclude extravasation by retrograde filling. If this exists, embolization through the second limb is carried out until cessation of extravasation is achieved.

In certain patients without angiographic evidence of contrast extravasation into the gastroduodenal lumen or other vascular anomaly, such as a pseudoaneurysm, neovascularity, or arteriovenous malformation, empirical or blind embolization is achieved based on conclusive endoscopic identification of the source of bleeding. Embolization of both the proximal and distal parts of the pseudoaneurysm should be done to prevent collateral filling. Embolization of the pseudoaneurysm at both ends of feeding arteries must be done to prevent collateral formation.

Our Experience

We have performed coil embolization of large gastroduodenal pseudoaneurysms secondary to pancreatitis presenting as gastrointestinal bleeding with a 98 % success rate, 0.1 % minor complications and 0.1 % recurrence rate (Figs. 7.14, 7.15, 7.16, 7.17, 7.18, 7.19, 7.20, 7.21, 7.22, 7.23, 7.24, and 7.25).

Tumor Embolization

Hepatocellular carcinoma (HCC) does not occur in a healthy liver. It usually develops in the setting of chronic hepatitis/cirrhosis viral hepatitis, alcohol abuse, and/or non-alcoholic steatohepatitis and frequently recurs after primary treatment due to the underlying liver disease [67, 68].

Transarterial chemoembolization (TACE) has been widely performed as a treatment for multifocal HCC in patients in whom curative treatment is difficult to perform [69].

According to the several staging systems for HCC, TACE is recommended only for large tumors (more than 3 cm) or multiple tumors (more than 4). However, in real clinical conditions, TACE is selected even for single HCCs in which it is difficult to perform surgical resection or locoregional treatment due to systemic co-morbidities or anatomical problems [70, 71].

TACE induces tumor necrosis through “starvation tactics”. It takes advantage of the fact that advanced HCCs are fed only by the hepatic artery and is intended to embolize the distal portion of the hepatic artery. The liver receives blood from the portal vein and hepatic artery at a ratio of 3:1 in the normal liver. Although this ratio varies in cirrhosis, the cirrhotic liver still receives blood flow from both of these vessels. In contrast, classical HCC (moderately-differentiated type) tumors receive nutritional blood flow through the hepatic artery only, and do not depend on portal vein blood flow.

Embolization using adriamycin or mitomycin C and gelfoam has been carried out since the first half of the 1980s. Intraarterial injection of lipiodol with anti-cancer drugs before embolic agent results in enhanced embolic effects [72, 73]. Through the use of microcatheter injection of lipiodol into the peripheral branches of the hepatic artery, segmental TACE/subsegmental TACE became a standard treatment. Segmental TACE/subsegmental TACE allows for strong locoregional embolization while stopping the portal blood flow, thereby improving the local treatment effects of TACE [7, 16].

Conventional TACE

Intra-tumor concentrations of drugs (particularly polymer drugs) are higher than those of normal tissue and blood due to the characteristics of blood vessels in solid tumors [72]. In hypervascular HCC, blood returns to the sinusoidal or portal vein as the tissue lacks associated lymphatics. This allows stasis of viscous liquid such as lipiodol in the sinusoidal or portal vein in or around HCCs.

It was observed that liver necrosis occurred following injection of lipiodol into the hepatic artery until it is visualized in the portal vein branch. Selective infusion of an anti-cancer drug/lipiodol mixture and an embolic agent (gelatin sponge) into tumor vessels is called conventional TACE.

The 1-year survival rate for TACE was reported as 44 %, [69] while segmental TACE had a 3-year survival rate of 67 % [74].

Ultra-Selective TACE

Ultra-selective TACE aims to achieve a local therapeutic effect through liver infarction. This technique involves insertion of a microcatheter selectively into a peripheral rather than subsegmental branch (subsubsegment artery), thereby wedging the tumor-feeding vessels, and then injecting lipiodol under high pressure into the tumor and surrounding sinusoids.

Ultra-selective TACE allows injection of lipiodol even into hypovascular lesions in well-differentiated HCC, and is reported to have a local control rate of 53.2 % in such cases [75].

Balloon Occlusive TACE

Due to extensive collateralization, when the embolization mixture is injected, backflow of blood occurs from portal vein and sinusoids. The hemodynamic changes caused by balloon occlusion reduce the arterial blood flow by closing the hepatic artery, thereby pushing lipiodol into the tumor under high pressure and enabling the drug to be intensively administered to the tumor, allowing for an enhanced therapeutic effect. In recent years, since microballoon catheters with small diameters have become more available, they have enhanced this delivery modality.

Platinum Complex Agents

In advanced HCC treatment, TACE functions as an efficient drug delivery system. Platinum complex agents are anti-cancer agents that cause DNA damage. Cisplatin, a first-generation platinum complex, and miriplatin, a third-generation platinum complex, are both used in the treatment of HCC [76–83]. Miriplatin is known to have less serious side effects and a lower incidence of renal failure compared to other platinum complex agents. Thus, miriplatin is considered to be suitable for repeat treatments, patients in whom cisplatin is contra-indicated and in elderly patients [84, 85].

Drug Eluting Bead

Unlike conventional gelatin sponges, the particle size of this material is uniform. Prediction of the level of embolism is straightforward, and a sustained embolic effect can be obtained. It is also possible to impregnate anti-cancer drugs into the beads, and the anti-tumor effect is improved due to the slow release of anti-cancer agents into the tumor.

The two types of widely used drug eluting beads are Hepasphere [86] and DC Bead [87].

DC Bead is derived from polyvinyl alcohol that is capable of impregnation of positively-charged drugs (*e.g.*, epirubicin, doxorubicin, or irinotecan). Its size is slightly decreased, and its hardness is increased by impregnation of anti-cancer drugs. Meanwhile, Hepasphere is derived from a polymer with high water absorption and can thus be impregnated with water-soluble anticancer agents. The size of Hepasphere increases following impregnation, it expands to about four times its size in the blood, and the resulting embolus is highly flexible and molds to the shape of the target vessel. Studies have demonstrated the superiority of these beads compared to TACE, however there is no statistically significant benefit in terms of mortality and morbidity.

The progress in therapeutic drugs, techniques and equipment has enabled enhanced therapeutic efficacy of TACE. It is necessary to individualize the treatment options for each patient.

Our Experience

We have performed chemoembolization for hepatic tumor in two patients using lipidol, cisplatin and gelfoam with success and 0 % complications (Figs. 7.28, 7.29, 7.30, 7.31, and 7.32).

Embolization of Glomus Tumors

Paragangliomas of the head and neck are tumors of the paraganglia which arise from neural crest progenitor cells [88]. The three most common sites for them are the carotid body, the jugular foramen, and the vagus nerve [89].

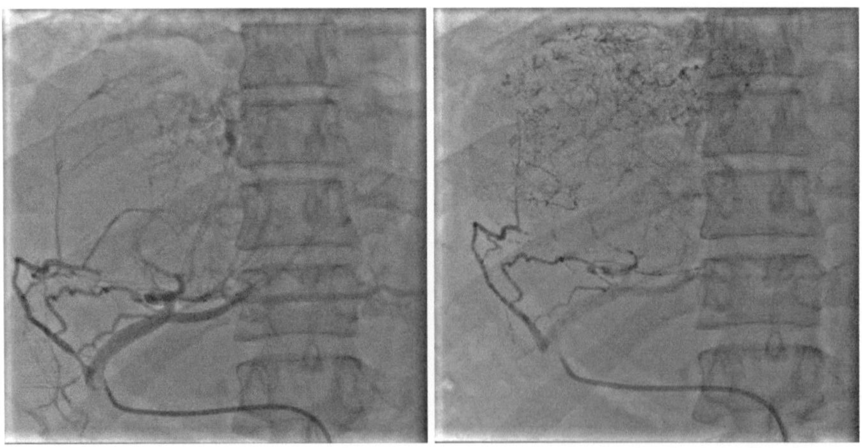

Figs. 7.28 and 7.29 Hepatic angiogram demonstrating increased vascularity and tumor blush

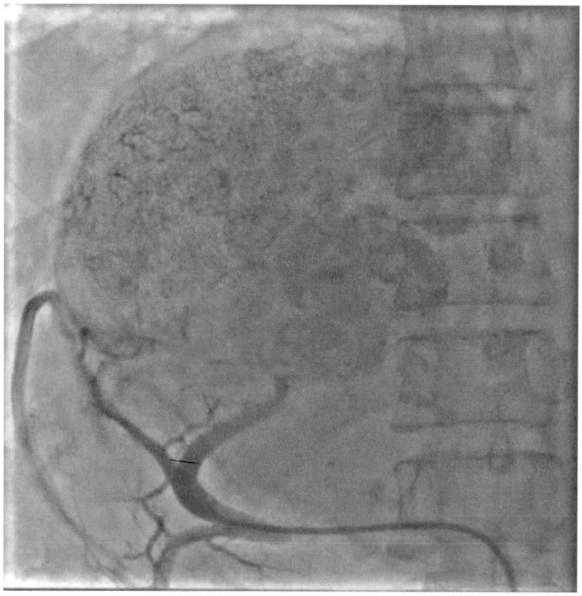

Fig. 7.30 Post-embolization angiogram demonstrating decrease in tumor vascularity with disappearance of the tumor blush

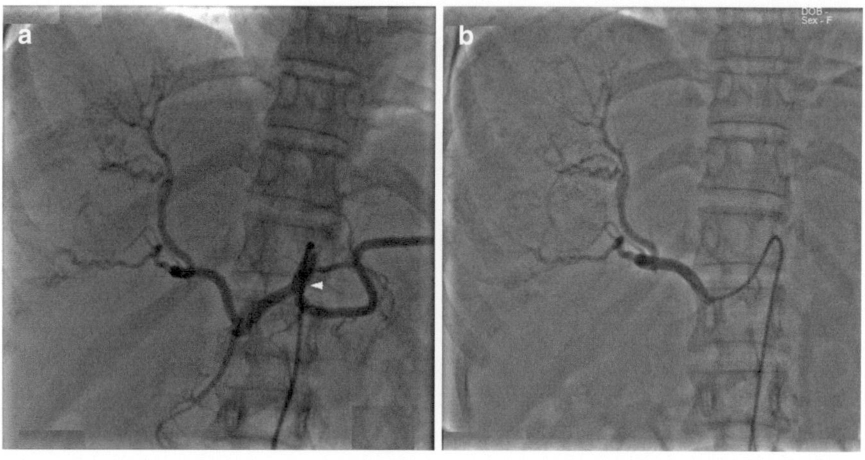

Fig. 7.31 (**a**) Coeliac angiography in a patient with inoperable malignant tumor of the liver. Note the sharp downward orientation of the coeliac artery (*arrowhead*) making it difficult for selective cannulation. A reverse curve (Simmons) catheter has been used (**b**) to selectively cannulate the hepatic artery for chemo-embolization. Tumor blush is noted in the right lobe of the liver

These tumors are highly vascular and the definitive treatment is surgical excision. Endovascular embolization prior to surgery is indicated to decrease vascularity of the tumor.

The classic angiographic appearance of a paraganglioma is that of a hypervascular mass with robust feeding arteries and an intense tumor blush [90, 91]. Across

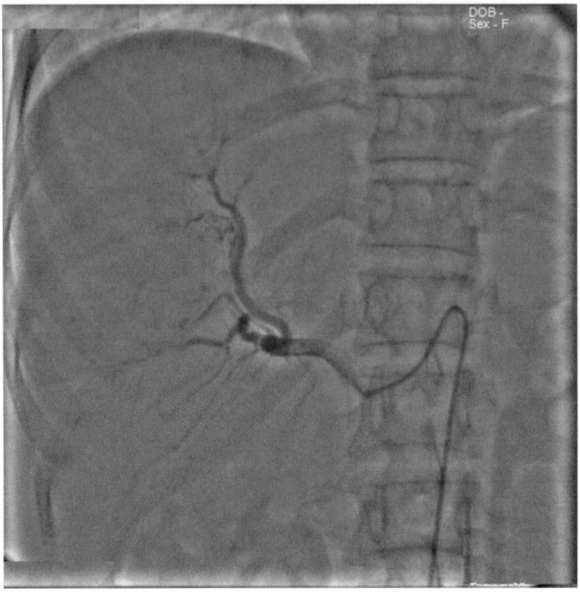

Fig. 7.32 Postembolization angiogram demonstrating decrease in tumor blush

most studies, the most common feeding vessel is the ascending pharyngeal artery [89, 92, 93] With tumor growth, other sources of arterial supply are usually recruited from any number of branches originating off of the ICA, ECA, or posterior circulation. Carotid body paragangliomas arise within the carotid body and characteristically splay the bifurcation of the common carotid artery [CCA] (Fig. 7.24) [94]. As the tumor enlarges, it may encase the ECA or ICA but normally does not compromise flow through them.

Vagal paragangliomas arise from glomus tissue and rests within the nodose ganglion. They are located just above the carotid bifurcation [95]. Angiographically, they are seen to compress the internal jugular vein and displace the carotid vessels anteriorly and medially.

Glomus jugulare tumors are defined as arising from within the jugular foramen [96]. Angiography reveals a tumor blush at the skull base with arterial feeders from the external carotid artery [ECA], internal carotid artery [ICA], and/or posterior circulation.

Technical Details

A 5 Fr diagnostic catheter is then advanced into the CCA on the ipsilateral side of the tumor. A CCA injection is performed to ensure that there are no ECA to ophthalmic artery anastomoses present that could compromise the patient's vision during embolization. The diagnostic catheter is advanced into the ECA where angiography is performed to determine the arterial feeders of the tumor. After completion of the diagnostic angiogram, a microcatheter is placed through the diagnostic catheter and advanced into selective branches of the ECA where selective arteriograms may be performed for improved tumor visualization. Initially, smaller particle size (150–250 microns) of PVA is used for embolization. Particles are placed in 1 ml syringes which are then attached to the microcatheter and injected in pulses. If flow to the tumor does not diminish, larger particle sizes (up to 1000 microns) are incrementally selected until there is cessation of flow in the vessel. This is done for all branches which can accommodate the microcatheter. A finishing angiogram from the CCA is performed to evaluate the degree of embolization and ensure patency of the ICA circulation.

Complications

Complications of preoperative embolization vary [97, 98]. Minor complications include fever and facial pain which are attributed to tumor ischemia and are usually transient. Major complications such as stroke may occur with the accidental introduction of embolics into the vertebrobasilar system via the ECA or its anastomoses with the ICA. Cranial nerve palsies occur with inadvertent introduction of embolic material into the vessels which supply them or use of particles that are too small thereby preventing a meaningful anastomoses to them. Other documented risks include transient aphasia, carotid sinus syndrome, and catecholamine storm.

Our Experience

We have performed embolization of a carotid body paraganglionoma in two patients, with 100 % success rate, 0 % complication and significant tumor devascularization prior to surgery (Figs. 7.33, 7.34, 7.35, and 7.36).

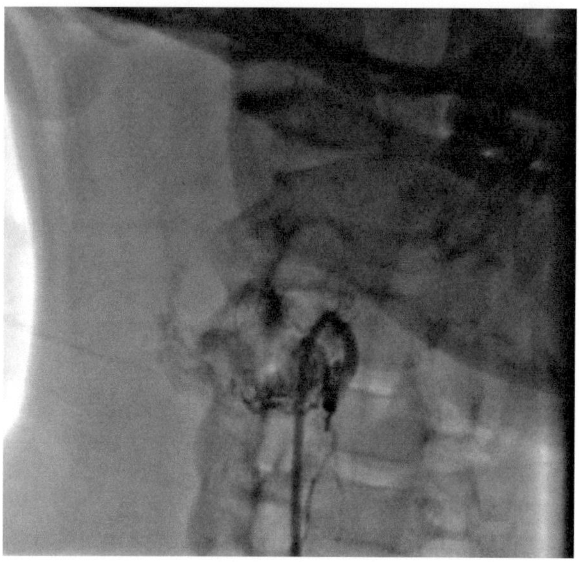

Fig. 7.33 Carotid angiogram demonstrating a carotid body paraganglionoma with increased vascularity

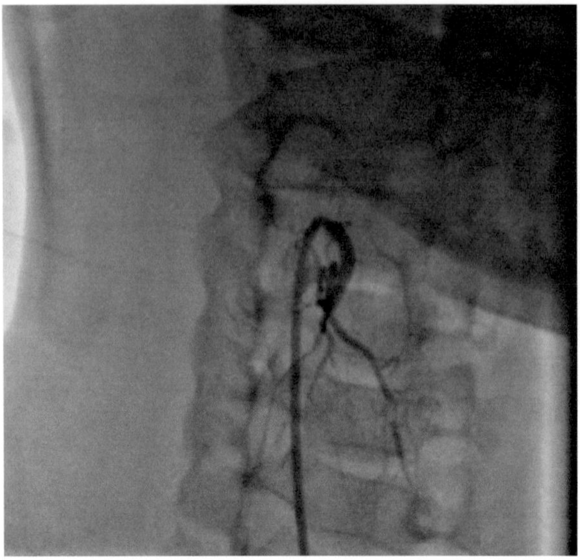

Fig. 7.34 Post-embolization angiogram demonstrating decreased vascularity of the tumor.

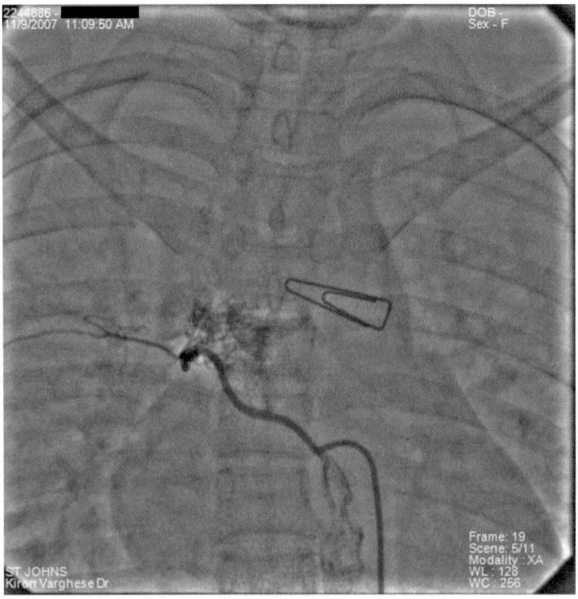

Fig. 7.35 Angiogram demonstrating a vertebral body AVM causing spinal cord compression

The embolization of paragangliomas using PVA prior to surgical resection is a safe and efficacious procedure that reduces operative blood loss and associated morbidity.

Complications can be significantly reduced by proper scrutiny of the pre-embolization angiogram which is a pre-requisite for all embolizations.

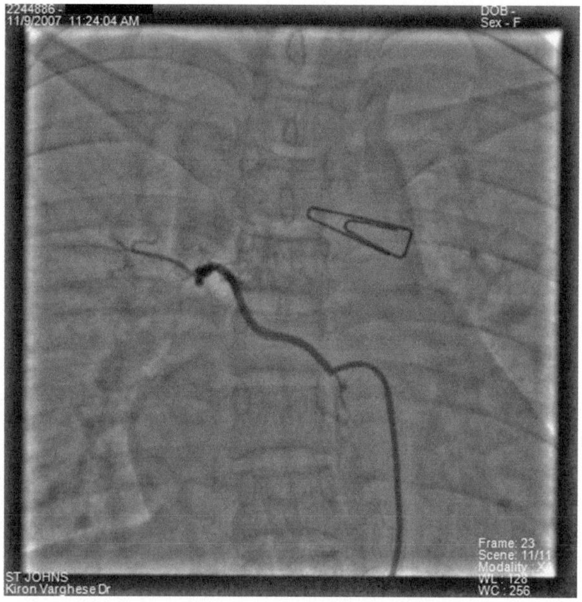

Fig. 7.36 Postembolization Angiogram demonstrating occlusion of the vertebral AVM

References

1. Seiffert A. Unterbindung der Arteria maxillaris interna. Zeitschrift fur Hals-, Nasen-, und Ohrenheilkunde. 1928;(22):323–9.
2. Sokoloff J, Wickbom I, McDonald D, Brahme F, Goergen TC, Goldberger LE. Therapeutic percutaneous embolization in intractable epistaxis. Radiology. 1974;111(2):285–7.
3. Schaitkin B, Strauss M, Houck JR. Epistaxis: medical versus surgical therapy: a comparison of efficacy, complications, and economic considerations. Laryngoscope. 1987;97(12):1392–6.
4. Small M, Murray JA, Maran AG. A study of patients with epistaxis requiring admission to hospital. Health Bull (Edinb). 1982;40(1):20–9.
5. Vitek J. Idiopathic intractable epistaxis: endovascular therapy. Radiology. 1991;181(1):113–6.
6. Fukutsuji K, Nishiike S, Aihara T, et al. Superselective angiographic embolization for intractable epistaxis. Acta Otolaryngol. 2008;128(5):556–60.
7. Ricci G, Molini E, Hamam M, et al. Treatment of severe epistaxis by superselective embolization: a review of 22 cases. Rev Laryngol Otol Rhinol (Bord). 2004;125(4):247–51.
8. Strutz JSM, Schumacher M. Uncontrollable epistaxis. Angiographic localization and embolization. Arch Otolaryngol Head Neck Surg. 1990;116(6):697–9.
9. Oguni T, Korogi Y, Yasunaga T, et al. Superselective embolisation for intractable idiopathic epistaxis. Br J Radiol. 2000;73(875):1148–53.
10. Mahmoud NA. Traumatic aneurysm of the internal carotid artery and epistaxis. (Review of literature and report of a case). J Laryngol Otol. 1979;93(6):629–56.
11. Karkanevatos A, Karkos PD, Karagama YG, Foy P. Massive recurrent epistaxis from non-traumatic bilateral intracavernous carotid artery aneurysms. Eur Arch Otorhinolaryngol. 2005; 262(7):546–9.
12. Elden L, Montanera W, Terbrugge K, et al. Angiographic embolization for the treatment of epistaxis: a review of 108 cases. Otolaryngol Head Neck Surg. 1994;111(1):44–50.
13. Wehrli M, Lieberherr U, Valavanis A. Superselective embolization for intractable epistaxis: experiences with 19 patients. Clin Otolaryngol Allied Sci. 1988;13(6):415–20.

14. Strach K, Schröck A, Wilhelm K, et al. Endovascular treatment of epistaxis: indications, management, and outcome. Cardiovasc Intervent Radiol. 2011;34(6):1190–8.
15. Cohen JE, Moscovici S, Gomori JM, Eliashar R, Weinberger J, Itshayek E. Selective endovascular embolization for refractory idiopathic epistaxis is a safe and effective therapeutic option: technique, complications, and outcomes. J Clin Neurosci. 2012;19(5):687–90.
16. Kendall B, Moseley I. Therapeutic embolisation of the external carotid arterial tree. J Neurol Neurosurg Psychiatry. 1977;40(10):937–50.
17. Smith TP. Embolization in the external carotid artery. J Vasc Interv Radiol. 2006;17(12): 1897–912; quiz 1913.
18. Metson R, Hanson DG. Bilateral facial nerve paralysis following arterial embolization for epistaxis. Otolaryngol Head Neck Surg. 1983;91(3):299–303.
19. Santaolalla F, Araluce I, Zabala A, López A, Garay M, Sanchez JM. Efficacy of selective percutaneous embolization for the treatment of intractable posterior epistaxis and juvenile nasopharyngeal angiofibroma (JNA). Acta Otolaryngol. 2009;129(12):1456–62.
20. Mok JS, Marshall JN, Chan M, van Hasselt CA. Percutaneous embolization to control intractable epistaxis in nasopharyngeal carcinoma. Head Neck. 1999;21(3):211–6.
21. Low YM, Goh YH. Endovascular treatment of epistaxis in patients irradiated for nasopharyngeal carcinoma. Clin Otolaryngol Allied Sci. 2003;28(3):244–7.
22. Celik SE, Celik S, Kelten B. Extraduralmeningioma presenting with severe epistaxis: a case report and review of the literature. J Neurosurg Sci. 2009;53(1):27–30.
23. Cloutier T, Pons Y, Blancal JP, et al. Juvenile nasopharyngeal angiofibroma: does the external approach still make sense? Otolaryngol Head Neck Surg. 2012;147(5):958–63.
24. Hodges JM, McDevitt AS, El-Sayed Ali AI, Sebelik ME. Juvenile nasopharyngeal angiofibroma: current treatment modalities and future considerations. Indian J Otolaryngol Head Neck Surg. 2010;62(3):236–47.
25. Gurney TA, Dowd CF, Murr AH. Embolization for the treatment of idiopathic posterior epistaxis. Am J Rhinol. 2004;18(5):335–9.
26. Willems PWA, Farb RI, Agid R. Endovascular treatment of epistaxis. AJNR Am J Neuroradiol. 2009;30(9):1637–45.
27. Sakamoto T, Yagi K, Hiraide A, et al. Transcatheter embolization in the treatment of massive bleeding due to maxillofacial injury. J Trauma. 1988;28(6):840–3.
28. Duggan CA, Brylski JR. Angiographic demonstration of bleeding in intractable traumatic epistaxis. Radiology. 1970;97(3):605–6.
29. Sumiyoshi K, Tsuneyoshi M, Enjoji M. M Y O S I T I S O S S I F I C A N S a clinicopathologic study of 21 cases. Acta Pathol Jpn. 1985;35(5):1109–22.
30. Oz BB, Boneh A. Myositis ossificans progressive: a 10-year follow-up on a patient treated with etidronate disodium. Acta Paediatr. 1994;83:1332–4.
31. Hendifar AE, Dorothy J, Daniel GA. Myositis ossificans: a case report arthritis & rheumatism. Arthritis Care Res. 2005;53(5):793–5.
32. Mann EG. Short report myositis ossificans in medieval London. Int J Osteoarchaeol. 1993;3:223–6.
33. Kohout MP, Hansen M, Pribaz JJ, Mulliken JB. Arteriovenous malformations of the head and neck: natural history and management. Plast Reconstr Surg. 1998;102(3):643–54.
34. Richter GT, Suen JY. Clinical course of arteriovenous malformations of the head and neck: a case series. Otolaryngol Head Neck Surg. 2010;142(2):184–90.
35. Bradley JP, Zide BM, Berenstein A, Longaker MT. Large arteriovenous malformations of the face: aesthetic results with recurrence control. Plast Reconstr Surg. 1999;103(2):351–61.
36. Ziyeh S, Strecker R, Berlis A, Weber J, Klisch J, Mader I. Dynamic 3D MR angiography of intra- and extracranial vascular malformations at 3T: a technical note. AJNR Am J Neuroradiol. 2005;26(3):630–4.
37. Tao Q, Lv B, Bhatia KSS, Qiao B, Zheng CQ, Chen ZF. Three-dimensional CT angiography for the diagnosis and assessment of arteriovenous malformations in the oral and maxillofacial region. J Cranio-Maxillofac Surg. 2010;38(1):32–7.

38. Thiex R, Wu I, Mulliken JB, Greene AK, Rahbar R, Orbach DB. Safety and clinical efficacy of onyx for embolization of extracranial head and neck vascular anomalies. AJNR Am J Neuroradiol. 2011;32(6):1082–6.
39. Richter GT, Suen J, North PE, James CA, Waner M, Buckmiller LM. Arteriovenous malformations of the tongue: a spectrum of disease. Laryngoscope. 2007;117(2):328–35.
40. Arat A, Cil BE, Vargel I, et al. Embolization of high-flow craniofacial vascular malformations with Onyx. AJNR Am J Neuroradiol. 2007;28(7):1409–14.
41. Fearon JA. Discussion: extracranial arteriovenous malformations: natural progression and recurrence after treatment. Plast Reconstr Surg. 2010;125(4):1195–6.
42. Visser A, Fitzjohn T, Tan ST. Surgical management of arteriovenous malformation. J Plast Reconstr Aesthet Surg. 2011;64(3):283–91.
43. Khurshid I, Downie GH. Pulmonary arteriovenous malformation: review. Postgrad Med J. 2002;78:191–7.
44. White Jr RI, Lynch-Nyhan A, Terry P, et al. Pulmonary arteriovenous malformations: technique and long-term of embolotherapy. Radiology. 1988;169:663–9.
45. Dutton JA, Jackson JE, Hughes JM, et al. Pulmonary arteriovenous malformations: results of treatment with coil embolization in 53 patients. AJR Am J Roentgenol. 1995;165: 1119–25.
46. Porteous ME, Burn J, Proctor SJ. Hereditary haemorrhagic telangiectasia: a clinical analysis. J Med Genet. 1992;29:527–30.
47. Faughnan ME, Lui YW, Wirth JA, et al. Diffuse pulmonary arteriovenous malformations: characteristics and prognosis. Chest. 2000;117:31–8.
48. Dinkel HP, Triller J. Pulmonary arteriovenous malformations: embolotheraphy with superselective coaxial catheter placement and filling of venous sac with Guglielmi detachable coils. Radiology. 2002;223:709–14.
49. Burke CM, Safai C, Nelson DP. Pulmonary arteriovenous malformations: a critical update. Am Rev Respir Dis. 1986;134:334–9.
50. Begbie ME, Wallace GMF, Shavlin CL. Hereditary haemorrhagic telangiectasia (Osler-Weber-Rendu syndrome): a view from the 21st century. Postgrad Med J. 2002;79:18–24.
51. Taylor BG, Cadgerill EM, Manferidi F, et al. Therapeutic embolization of the pulmonary artery in pulmonary arteriovenous fistula. Am J Med. 1978;64:360–5.
52. Haitjema TJ, Overtoom TT, Westermann CJ, Lammers JW. Embolization of pulmonary arteriovenous malformations: results and follow up in 32 patients. Thorax. 1995;50:719–23.
53. White AF, Baum S, Buranasiri S. Aneurysms secondary to pancreatitis. AJR Am J Roentgenol. 1976;127:393–6. Epub 1976/09/01.
54. Chong WW, Tan SG, Htoo MM. Endovascular treatment of gastroduodenal artery aneurysm. Asian Cardiovasc Thorac Ann. 2008;16(1):68–72. Epub 2008/02/05.
55. Morita Y, Kawamura N, Saito H, Shinohara M, Irie G, Okushiba S, et al. [Diagnosis and embolotherapy of aneurysm of the gastroduodenal artery]. Rinsho Hoshasen Clin Radiography. 1988;33(5):555–61. Epub 1988/05/01.
56. Matsuzaki Y, Inoue T, Kuwajima K, Ito Y, Okauchi Y, Kondo H, et al. Aneurysm of the gastroduodenal artery. Int Med (Tokyo, Japan). 1998;37(11):930–3. Epub 1998/12/30.
57. Shanley CJ, Shah NL, Messina LM. Uncommon splanchnic artery aneurysms: pancreaticoduodenal, gastroduodenal, superior mesenteric, inferior mesenteric, and colic. Ann Vasc Surg. 1996;10(5):506–15. Epub 1996/09/01.
58. Deterling Jr RA. Aneurysm of the visceral arteries. J Cardiovasc Surg. 1971;12(4):309–22. Epub 1971/07/01.
59. Kueper MA, Ludescher B, Koenigsrainer I, Kirschniak A, Mueller K, Wiskirchen J, et al. Successful coil embolization of a ruptured gastroduodenal artery aneurysm. Vasc Endovascular Surg. 2007;41(6):568–71. Epub 2008/01/02.
60. Gouny P, Fukui S, Aymard A, Decaix B, Mory H, Merland JJ, et al. Aneurysm of the gastroduodenal artery associated with stenosis of the superior mesenteric artery. Ann Vasc Surg. 1994;8(3):281–4. Epub 1994/05/01.

61. Quandalle P, Chambon JP, Marache P, Saudemont A, Maes B. Pancreaticoduodenal artery aneurysms associated with celiac axis stenosis: report of two cases and review of the literature. Ann Vasc Surg. 1990;4(6):540–5. Epub 1990/11/01.
62. Bergert H, Hinterseher I, Kersting S, Leonhardt J, Bloomenthal A, Saeger HD. Management and outcome of hemorrhage due to arterial pseudoaneurysms in pancreatitis. Surgery. 2005;137(3):323–8. Epub 2005/03/05.
63. Lee PC, Rhee RY, Gordon RY, Fung JJ, Webster MW. Management of splenic artery aneurysms: the significance of portal and essential hypertension. J Am Coll Surg. 1999;189(5):483–90. Epub 1999/11/05.
64. Moore E, Matthews MR, Minion DJ, Quick R, Schwarcz TH, Loh FK, et al. Surgical management of peripancreatic arterial aneurysms. J Vasc Surg Off Publ Soc Vasc Surg Int Soc Cardiovasc Surg North Am Chapter. 2004;40(2):247–53. Epub 2004/08/07.
65. Rowsell C, Moore TL, Streutker CJ. Aneurysm of the gastroduodenal artery presenting as a bleeding duodenal ulcer. Clin Gastroenterology Hepatol Off Clin Pract J Am Gastroenterological Assoc. 2006;4(10):xxviii. Epub 2006/06/08.
66. Skok P, Sinkovic A. Acute hemorrhage into the peritoneal cavity—a complication of chronic pancreatitis with pseudocyst: a case report from clinical practice. Hepatogastroenterology. 1999;46(25):518–21. Epub 1999/05/06.
67. Ikeda K, Kobayashi M, Kawamura Y, Imai N, Seko Y, Hirakawa M, Hosaka T, Sezaki H, Akuta N, Saitoh S, Suzuki F, Suzuki Y, Arase Y, Kumada H. Stage progression of small hepatocellular carcinoma after radical therapy: comparisons of radiofrequency ablation and surgery using the Markov model. Liver Int. 2011;31:692–9. [PMID: 21457441 doi:10.1111/j.1478-3231.2011.02480.x].
68. Ikeda K, Kawamura Y, Kobayashi M, Fukushima T, Sezaki H, Hosaka T, Akuta N, Saitoh S, Suzuki F, Suzuki Y, Arase Y, Kumada H. Prevention of disease progression with anti-inflammatory therapy in patients with HCV-related cirrhosis: a Markov model. Oncology. 2014;86:295–302. [PMID: 24924385 doi:10.1159/000357713].
69. Yamada R, Sato M, Kawabata M, Nakatsuka H, Nakamura K, Takashima S. Hepatic artery embolization in 120 patients with unresectable hepatoma. Radiology. 1983;148:397–401. [PMID: 6306721 doi:10.1148/radiology.148.2.6306721].
70. Bruix J, Sherman M. Management of hepatocellular carcinoma: an update. Hepatology. 2011;53:1020–2. [PMID: 21374666 doi:10.1002/hep.24199].
71. Arii S, Sata M, Sakamoto M, Shimada M, Kumada T, Shiina S, Yamashita T, Kokudo N, Tanaka M, Takayama T, Kudo M. Management of hepatocellular carcinoma: report of consensus meeting in the 45th Annual Meeting of the Japan Society of Hepatology (2009). Hepatol Res. 2010;40:667–85. [PMID:20633193 doi:10.1111/j.1872-034X.2010.00673.x].
72. Matsumura Y, Maeda H. A new concept for macromolecular therapeutics in cancer chemotherapy: mechanism of tumoritropic accumulation of proteins and the antitumor agent smancs. Cancer Res. 1986;46:6387–92. [PMID: 2946403.
73. Uchida H, Ohishi H, Matsuo N, Nishimine K, Ohue S, Nishimura Y, Maeda M, Yoshioka T. Transcatheter hepatic segmental arterial embolization using lipiodol mixed with an anticancer drug and Gelfoam particles for hepatocellular carcinoma. Cardiovasc Intervent Radiol. 1990;13:140–5. [PMID: 2171772].
74. Takayasu K, Muramatsu Y, Maeda T, Iwata R, Furukawa H, Muramatsu Y, Moriyama N, Okusaka T, Okada S, Ueno H. Targeted transarterial oily chemoembolization for small foci of hepatocellular carcinoma using a unified helical CT and angiography system: analysis of factors affecting local recurrence and survival rates. AJR Am J Roentgenol. 2001;176:681–8. [PMID: 11222205 doi:10.2214/ajr.176.3.1760681].
75. Miyayama S, Matsui O, Yamashiro M, Ryu Y, Takata H, Takeda T, Aburano H, Shigenari N. Iodized oil accumulation in the hypovascular tumor portion of early-stage hepatocellular carcinoma after ultraselective transcatheter arterial chemoembolization. Hepatol Int. 2007;1:451–9. [PMID:19669342 doi:10.1007/s12072-007-9030-5].
76. Sahara S, Tanihata H, Sato M, Kawai N, Takasaka I, Minamiguchi H, Nakai M, Sonomura T. Effects of hepatic artery chemoembolization using cisplatin-lipiodol suspension with

gelatin sponge particles on swine liver. J Vasc Interv Radiol. 2009;20:1359–64. [PMID: 19695901 doi:10.1016/j.jvir.2009.06.028].

77. Kawaoka T, Aikata H, Takaki S, Katamura Y, Hiramatsu A, Waki K, Takahashi S, Hieda M, Toyota N, Ito K, Chayama K. Transarterial infusion chemotherapy using cisplatin-lipiodol suspension with or without embolization for unresectable hepatocellular carcinoma. Cardiovasc Intervent Radiol. 2009;32:687–94. [PMID: 19444503 doi:10.1007/s00270-009-9570-2].
78. Osuga K, Arai Y, Anai H, Takeuchi Y, Aramaki T, Sugihara E, Yamamoto T, Inaba Y, Ganaha F, Seki H, Sadaoka S, Sato M, Kobayashi T, Kodama Y, Inoh S, Yamakado K. Phase I/II multicenter study of transarterial chemoembolization with a cisplatin fine powder and porous gelatin particles for unresectable hepatocellular carcinoma: Japan Interventional Radiology in Oncology Study Group Study 0401. J Vasc Interv Radiol. 2012;23:1278–85. [PMID: 22922041 doi:10.1016/j.jvir.2012.06.028].
79. Kim HC, Lee JH, Chung JW, Kang B, Yoon JH, Kim YJ, Lee HS, Jae HJ, Park JH. Transarterial chemoembolization with additional cisplatin infusion for hepatocellular carcinoma invading the hepatic vein. J Vasc Interv Radiol. 2013;24:274–83. [PMID: 23369561 doi:10.1016/j.jvir.2012.11.002].
80. Kawamura Y, Ikeda K, Fukushima T, Seko Y, Hara T, Sezaki H, Hosaka T, Akuta N, Kobayashi M, Saitoh S, Suzuki F, Suzuki Y, Arase Y, Kumada H. What is the most effective drug delivery system for cisplatin during the treatment of hepatic tumors with single-session transcatheter chemotherapy? A Pilot Study. Gut Liver. 2013;7:576–84. [PMID: 24073316 doi:10.5009/gnl.2013.7.5.576].
81. Imai N, Ikeda K, Seko Y, Kawamura Y, Sezaki H, Hosaka T, Akuta N, Kobayashi M, Saitoh S, Suzuki F, Suzuki Y, Arase Y, Kumada H. Previous chemoembolization response after transcatheter arterial chemoembolization (TACE) can predict the anti-tumor effect of subsequent TACE with miriplatin in patients with recurrent hepatocellular carcinoma. Oncology. 2011;80:188–94. [PMID: 21709428 doi:10.1159/000328749].
82. Okusaka T, Kasugai H, Ishii H, Kudo M, Sata M, Tanaka K, Shioyama Y, Chayama K, Kumada H, Yoshikawa M, Seki T, Saito H, Hayashi N, Shiratori K, Okita K, Sakaida I, Honda M, Kusumoto Y, Tsutsumi T, Sakata K. A randomized phase II trial of intra-arterial chemotherapy using SM-11355 (Miriplatin) for hepatocellular carcinoma. Invest New Drugs. 2012;30:2015–25. [PMID: 22187203 doi:10.1007/s10637-011-9776-4].
83. Imai Y, Chikayama T, Nakazawa M, Watanabe K, Ando S, Mizuno Y, Yoshino K, Sugawara K, Hamaoka K, Fujimori K, Inao M, Nakayama N, Oka M, Nagoshi S, Mochida S. Usefulness of miriplatin as an anticancer agent for transcatheter arterial chemoembolization in patients with unresectable hepatocellular carcinoma. J Gastroenterol. 2011; Epub ahead of print. [PMID: 21976133 doi:10.1007/s00535-011-0475-x].
84. Imai N, Ikeda K, Kawamura Y, Sezaki H, Hosaka T, Akuta N, Kobayashi M, Saitoh S, Suzuki F, Suzuki Y, Arase Y, Kumada H. Transcatheter arterial chemotherapy using miriplatinlipiodol suspension with or without embolization for unresectable hepatocellular carcinoma. Jpn J Clin Oncol. 2012;42:175–82. [PMID: 22210921 doi:10.1093/jjco/hyr189].
85. Imai N, Ikeda K, Seko Y, Kawamura Y, Sezaki H, Hosaka T, Akuta N, Kobayashi M, Saitoh S, Suzuki F, Suzuki Y, Arase Y, Kumada H. Transcatheter arterial chemotherapy with miriplatin for hepatocellular carcinoma patients with chronic renal failure: report of three cases. Gut Liver. 2013;7:246–51. [PMID: 23560163 doi:10.5009/gnl.2013.7.2.246].
86. Grosso M, Vignali C, Quaretti P, Nicolini A, Melchiorre F, Gallarato G, Bargellini I, Petruzzi P, Massa Saluzzo C, Crespi S, Sarti I. Transarterial chemoembolization for hepatocellular carcinoma with drug-eluting microspheres: preliminary results from an Italian multicentre study. Cardiovasc Intervent Radiol. 2008;31:1141–9. [PMID: 18696150 doi:10.1007/s00270-008-9409-2].
87. Lewis AL, Gonzalez MV, Lloyd AW, Hall B, Tang Y, Willis SL, Leppard SW, Wolfenden LC, Palmer RR, StratfordPW. DC bead: in vitro characterization of a drug-delivery device for transarterial chemoembolization. J Vasc Interv Radiol. 2006;17:335–42. [PMID: 16517780 doi:10.1097/01.RVI.0000195323.46152.B3].

88. Boedeker CC, Ridder GJ, Schipper J. Paragangliomas of the head and neck: diagnosis and treatment. Fam Cancer. 2005;4:55–9.
89. Valavanis A. Preoperative embolization of the head and neck: indications, patient selection, goals, and precautions. AJNR Am J Neuroradiol. 1986;7:943–52.
90. Myssiorek D. Head and neck paragangliomas: an overview. Otolaryngol Clin North Am. 2001;34:829–36.
91. Wasserman PG, Savargaonkar P. Paragangliomas: classification, pathology, and differential diagnosis. Otolaryngol Clin North Am. 2001;34:845–62.
92. Tikkakoski T, Luotonen J, Leinonen S, et al. Preoperative embolization in the management of neck paragangliomas. Laryngoscope. 1997;107:821–6.
93. Smith RF, Shetty PC, Reddy DJ. Surgical treatment of carotid paragangliomas presenting unusual technical difficulties. The value of preoperative embolization. J Vasc Surg. 1988; 7:631–7.
94. Luna-Ortiz K, Rascon-Ortiz M, Villavicencio-Valencia V, et al. Carotid body tumors: review of a 20-year experience. Oral Oncol. 2005;41:56–61.
95. Davidson J, Gullane P. Glomus vagale tumors. Otolaryngol Head Neck Surg. 1988;99:66–70.
96. Jackson CG. Glomus tympanicum and glomus jugulare tumors. Otolaryngol Clin North Am. 2001;34:941–70.
97. Persky MS, Setton A, Niimi Y, et al. Combined endovascular and surgical treatment of head and neck paragangliomas–a team approach. Head Neck. 2002;24:423–31.
98. Tasar M, Yetiser S. Glomus tumors: therapeutic role of selective embolization. J Craniofac Surg. 2004;15:497–505.

Index

© Springer International Publishing Switzerland 2017
K. Varghese, S. Adhyapak, *Therapeutic Embolization*,
DOI 10.1007/978-3-319-42494-1

MIX
Papier aus verantwortungsvollen Quellen
Paper from responsible sources
FSC® C105338

If you have any concerns about our products,
you can contact us on
ProductSafety@springernature.com

In case Publisher is established outside the EU,
the EU authorized representative is:
Springer Nature Customer Service Center GmbH
Europaplatz 3, 69115 Heidelberg, Germany

Printed by Libri Plureos GmbH
in Hamburg, Germany